HEPATITIS C, CURED

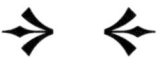

Johnny Delirious

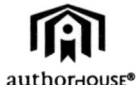

AuthorHouse™
1663 Liberty Drive, Suite 200
Bloomington, IN 47403
www.authorhouse.com
Phone: 1-800-839-8640

© *2009 Johnny Delirious. All rights reserved.*

No part of this book may be reproduced, stored in a retrieval system, or transmitted by any means without the written permission of the author.

First published by AuthorHouse 2/2/2009

ISBN: 978-1-4389-4547-7 (sc)
ISBN: 978-1-4389-4548-4 (dj)

Printed in the United States of America
Bloomington, Indiana

This book is printed on acid-free paper.

Based on true experiences of its author, the entire content of this book is intended to provide useful anecdotal health information to the reader and to the public. All material contained herein is for informational purposes only and is not a substitute for medical diagnosis, advice, or treatment for any specific and/or general medical condition. Every reader should seek expert medical care and consult his/her own physicians for any specific health issues. The author does not recommend or endorse any specific tests, procedures, regimens, advice or other information presented in these contents, and specifically disclaims all responsibility for any liability, loss, or risk, personal or otherwise, which is incurred as a consequence, directly or indirectly, of the use or application of any of the procedures and/or regimens depicted in these contents.

This book is dedicated to everyone living on planet Earth who suffers from Hepatitis.

Introduction------Diagnosis

1   Fort Walton
2   Denial
3   Hepatitis High
4   Another Statistic
5   The Establishment
6   Acceptance
7   Mexico Squared
8   Going Natural
9   Laboratory Life
10   War
11   The Zapper
12   Peace
13   Popeye
14   Bluto
15   Fanatic
16   The Rule
17   Gerson Clinic
18   Depression
19   Rife
20   Anticipation
21   Top Gun
22   Liver = Health
23   Riders of the Storm
24   Walk the Line

Epilogue-------Inside Job

Diagnosis

"Eight months."

Few spoken words had ever delivered more impact than those two simple ones did. Understandable, since it was my doctor who said them. She was only trying to answer an uncomplicated question; one that I was admittedly more than a little afraid to ask.

But I asked. And she answered. A bit too matter-of-factly, for my taste. I was going to be one of the unlucky ones, thank you very much.

But wait. Hold on a second. I had *already* been unlucky more than once, when I was infected with both hepatitis A and B in high school. True, I had *survived* those episodes, but what the heck for? So I could die of Hepatitis C twenty-two years later?

Sorry. Twenty-two years and *eight months* later.

Not fair, why me, what cruel justice is this? How did God decide it was my turn again?

A thing or two will cross a man's mind when he learns he'll be on the wrong side of the grass in less than a year. Like most mortals, I had never really thought all that much about death. Thirty-nine is not so ripe an age that one should be *expected* to think about it, right?

Well, I was thinking about it now, for sure. And the Doc was droning on about treatment options and what not, but I wasn't listening to her.

I was thinking about dying.

Before the Doc's unceremonious announcement, I had already known that I had "Non-A, non B" hepatitis. I had known, too, that things were getting serious. The jaundice, the fatigue, loss of appetite and weight, even the way the veins looked in my hands. All clues to the progress the disease was making in its effort to take me apart.

Current estimates suggest that over 3,000,000 Americans currently have chronic hepatitis C. And the Center for Disease Control puts the number of people in the US that have ever been infected with "C" at 1.6% of the population.

Put another way, if 200 people make up the congregation of your church on any given Sunday, which three of them have had hepatitis C?

Up to fifty thousand people die worldwide of hepatitis C every year, eight to ten thousand of them right here in the United States.

Kind of a sobering thought.

So now, with the Doc chattering away about liver transplants, clinical trials, interferon, and drug cocktails, I was thinking about *dying*.

In eight months.

Fort Walton Beach

Western Florida, for the most part, is not so bad a place to grow up.

With a population hovering around 20,000, Fort Walton Beach, Florida, is probably best known for being in the thick of the Air Force and Navy bases that dot the panhandle. The Naval Air Station in Pensacola is only 40 miles away from Fort Walton, and the town directly borders Eglin Air Force base and Hurlburt Field.

Among others, Eglin hosts the 33rd Air Combat Command fighter wing and as one of the larger US bases (in terms of land mass) it is also home to cooperative military exercises and bomb ordinance testing. In fact, the now-famous "Mother of All Bombs" was tested here at Eglin Air Force base, before the 20,000-pound monster could unleash its wrath on real targets in combat theaters.

Living near a military base was kind of good and bad at the same time. It meant that you could make new friends easily enough, no doubt. On the other hand, you were constantly *making* new friends because the other new friends you just made were always leaving for a different base in a different state.

Or a different country, for that matter.

Not too many famous people hail from my home town, but we can claim a few. Jason Elam, the guy who kicked field goals for the Denver Broncos and Astronaut Richard Covey are from Fort Walton. And we always had our share of beautiful women just about everywhere in Florida, but Fort Walton is also home to Carolyn Murphy, the well-known supermodel born here in 1973.[1]

---

[1] http://en.wikipedia.org/wiki/Fort_Walton_Beach,_Florida

Our fine city was named after the Camp Walton Civil War site occupied by the Walton Guards during the war. It was permanently so named in 1932 after the discovery of a buried Civil War cannon in the heart of what is presently the downtown area of the city.[2]

Most of my youth was spent in and around Fort Walton Beach. The sugar-white beaches of the Emerald Coast, from Pensacola to Panama City, and the inland bayous nearby are, to me, some of the finest gifts God has ever given to us.

In my earliest years, I was active in the Episcopal Church as an Acolyte (much like an altar boy). Bible class was central to my development as a person. So were the activities our church supported and encouraged for the youth of the congregation.

One such activity was the regular occurrence of musical jamborees. Back in the 50's and 60's, Western Florida was one of many stops that church and gospel singing groups made on their tours of the country. In particular, the Halleluiah Hay Ride troop visited Tower Beach, which my two older sisters took me along as a little kid. A little kid whose eyes swelled to the size of saucers when he got to see the King himself, Elvis Presley, up there singing as part of a large gospel chorus. He would have been just 24 then, and I was only seven. I guess a lot of people have forgotten the heavy influence that gospel music had on what would eventually become rock 'n roll.

I haven't forgotten it. For me, those jamborees and gospel concerts were some of the best times of my life.

--

As the 1960's progressed, Fort Walton Beach became known as one of the country's fastest growing cities. The population exploded during this time, increasing seven-fold[3] while I moved from childhood to adolescence. This happened despite the arrival of oral contraceptives on the scene, the FDA having approved them early in the decade.

You could buy a nice 3-bedroom, 1-1/2 bath house on 13 acres for around $17,000 at the time, gas was 34 cents a gallon, and the average income for an American worker was under eight grand a year.[4]

---

[2] http://www.fwb.org/content.php?page=49
[3] http://www.fwb.org/content.php?page=49
[4] http://www.thepeoplehistory.com/1968.html

During this time, Eglin and its sister base at Hurlburt Field also continued to grow, both of them bringing our town the typical high turnover of fresh Air Force brats to join us in school. Like I said, it seemed that making new friends was never really a problem.

Or so I thought.

Denial

The drive back to my brother's house from the University of Mississippi Medical Center in Jackson, MS takes no more than 20 minutes. Plenty of time for a man to think about things he ordinarily wouldn't; things like liver transplant donors, second opinions, and being really, really mad at God.

Moving along at 45 mph, one thought that occurred to me was I needed to stop by the grocery store, it was time to pick up a couple jugs of fresh spring water.

At this, I laughed out loud. Such things seemed so trivial now.

It had been seven years since a different Doc right here in Jackson had broken the news that I had hepatitis all over again. This time it wasn't hep A or hep B; they were calling it "Non A-non B strain."

At the time I was just 32, a young man by anyone's standards, and one that had the typical list of action items required to achieve his own version of the American dream.

And now, those "action items" were starting to look a lot more like a bucket list. Was I really going to *die* some time in the next eight months? It didn't seem possible! I had been following doctor's orders the best I could, avoiding alcohol (almost all the time, anyway) and all the foods they told me would intensify the effects of the disease. I gave up everything from Twinkies to coffee to tap water, choosing health food and herbs instead.

All for nothing, quite apparently, despite my best efforts, the disease had taken a rather decisive grip on my liver.

Maybe I should have partied my way through these last seven years, it would've been better to go out with a bang.

On the other hand, what did any of these doctors really *know*? I mean no disrespect to the director of Gastroenterology at University Medical, but how could she be so sure that my case of "Non-A-non B" hepatitis constituted a death sentence? That is, unless I was willing to chuck my old liver out the door and start over with a new one. And how could she be so sure that a brand new liver wouldn't just get infected all over again anyway? After all, my track record in life thus far had included being something of a hepatitis magnet.

I had been no angel in my youth, like many of my peers; I had been a regular, red-blooded, all-American boy. Part of that meant that I did my share of chasing girls (not other boys, for the record). But I had been smart enough to avoid injecting narcotics into my bloodstream, so we can eliminate the most common cause of hepatitis from the list of possibilities in my case.

Whoops. "Cases," I meant, as in plural.

On the strength of a tissue biopsy report, this Gastroenterology specialist in Mississippi was saying this latest case had managed to ravage my liver to the point that only four percent of it remained free of scar tissue.

Not good.

When you have chronic liver disease, your functioning tissue is gradually destroyed over time. Scar tissue replaces normal liver tissue, in a progressive way that prevents regular blood flow to the organ itself. This leads to the complete breakdown of the tasks your liver is signed up to do, including the processing of nutrients, the dilution of poisons, and the production of crucial bodily fluids that you need to live.

This wonderful process is called "cirrhosis" of the liver. According to the National Institute of Diabetes, Digestive and Kidney Diseases, chronic liver disease is the seventh leading cause of death in the U.S. Things were beginning to look like it was going to be the cause of mine.

Heading south on US 51 outside of Jackson, MS, my focus was on anything but my driving. Just now, it was pointed in God's direction. Not in a very reverent way, either.

For most of my life, I had given God his due. I was a man of faith for all but a few of my rebellious teenage years, when I began to absorb a bit of influence from some of the non-believers in my life. But I can honestly say that I didn't come running back to God just because I got sick a few times. At around the age of 19, I got smart again and came to realize that 1) my dad really wasn't as dumb as I thought he was when I was a teenager; and 2) God is real and once I figured that out, I simply let Him back into my life.

Right now, though, I was kind of thinking about kicking him right back out.

"Screw that," I said out loud as the traffic thickened on highway 51. "I'll get another opinion."

If it turned out to be the same as the Doc from University Medical, I could always go back to blaming God then.

Hepatitis High

Bulletproof.

That's what you are when you're fifteen years old, wild and free-spirited, especially the way we were in the last years of the 1960's.

Touch-tone phones, manned spacecraft, satellite communications, color TV, the first mini-computer and feminism were all born during this turbulent time. The Dow was struggling to break the thousand-point barrier and America was struggling with the Vietnam War.

But my classmates at Choctawhatchee High School and me were rebellious and impervious to the threats and concerns of the time. We were sure we knew how to handle anything the world could throw at us, true *Catchers in the Rye*, unafraid of anything except growing up. We knew that growing older was inevitable, but we were doing our best to seize the spoils of youth and hold onto them hard.

There were the conventional distractions, of course. I was on the football team in my first years at high school. Tried out for the tennis team, too, but didn't focus hard enough to make a real go of it. I was more into waterskiing, scuba diving and all things Gulf-related as any true Florida boy would be.

The time I spent with athletics, however, did afford me the luxury of mixing well with just about any group of students I wanted to. I was known as a pretty agreeable guy, one who could get along with the jocks, the burnouts, or the geeks with equal ease and comfort. Never one to get into fist fights or cause trouble with my classmates, I was accepted by most everyone and blended well with all.

Because I was so good at "blending," I saw a lot of things, too many things, and some things I wish I had never seen or ever knew anything about. Some of it was really bad. Most of it was just a little bad.

Sometimes, when one particular friend who lived on the beach would see the surf swelling up, we'd grab our wetsuits and surfboards and leave the books at home. Skipping school in favor of surfing, fishing or waterskiing became somewhat common, and it didn't matter whether it was May or December. In Florida, you can enjoy the beach any time you like, as long as you're tough enough to handle the mean waves (when the Gulf wasn't flat) and the colder waters that winter brings.

When the moon was full, the tide was right and the redfish were biting, we had another handy excuse for cutting class. Destin, Florida is just 11 miles from Fort Walton Beach, and it has always called itself "The Luckiest Fishing Village in the World." In Destin, they pride themselves on the fact that you don't need a boat to experience some of the best sports fishing you can find. You can do it right off the beach pier, and it's best when the Pompano first show up in the spring.

There were times, though, when the fishing in Western Florida was not so lucky; particularly with shellfish.

The late '60's brought the first foreshadowing of hepatitis-related illnesses to our area. It came in the form of headlines in the paper, with reports such as *"Woman Hospitalized After Eating Contaminated Oysters."* Tainted seafood had become just one more thing for our parents to worry about in the swinging sixties.

Not us teenagers, though. We were bulletproof, remember? The kids in my group all had fake ID's, and we used them to sneak down to the oyster bars near the beach, where you could get all the oysters you could eat and all the beer you could drink for twelve bucks.

And drink we did. What was that famous saying by Paul Kantner of Jefferson Airplane?

*"If you can remember anything
about the sixties, you weren't really there."*

Well, I remember plenty about the sixties, but I was there. I was right there in the heart of it, along with my high school classmates, there with the ones that stayed in town year after year, and there with the ones who showed up new for a brief stop in Fort Walton on the way to the next Air Force or Navy town.

Over 40% of the class would have new faces in it when each new school year began. Many of those faces had felt the sun in other places far away from our little town in Florida. Military families that had spent time in countries like Guam, Germany, Korea, Okinawa, Hawaii, Vietnam, Thailand, and many others were now spending time with us. For the most part, I and those like me who were permanent fixtures in Fort Walton welcomed these new faces with open arms.

Some of those new faces, however, carried things with them that were not so welcome. Germs and afflictions foreign to our state became regular visitors when some of the military kids brought them along from another corner of the world. Maybe those military kids had gotten used to some of the bugs they carried, but us locals got sick often enough that it was clear to me we certainly weren't immune.

One ordinary day, the news arrived that a couple of guys in the group I hung around with most were sick with something more serious than the usual stuff. These were guys who had spent some time in Eastern Asia, and when we heard they were sick, we naturally attributed it to germs they had lugged over from that part of the planet.

But then I got sick, too.

The conventional wisdom says that you can get hepatitis A from transmission by human contact of one sort or another. Kissing, for example, or an infected person can sneeze in your face and you'll get a good case of hepatitis A just the same. So if someone had come in contact with the virus in another part of the world, they could easily transfer it to us innocent Floridians in any number of ways. At any rate, it's highly communicable.

Hepatitis B, on the other hand, requires a bit more "human contact" to move it about. It is most often transmitted by sexual contact or mixing of blood, as with drug users that share needles.

I had never used any drugs that required administration via a needle, so I knew that wasn't the cause for me. But within my circle of friends, there were four guys and three girls, each of whom we took turns going "steady" with. We were mixing friendship with people who had lived in remote countries, possibly tainted seafood, and sex with each other's girl friends in such a way that it became impossible to tell the true cause of our hepatitis cases.

Those of us who had thorough blood testing (I was one of them, thanks to my dad's medical clinic) showed that we had hepatitis B. Later, the CDC would find many replications of the disease, but this was 1970 and finding the exact strain required more testing, so at the time the ones related to local seafood could not be easily determined.

Like the common cold, hepatitis comes in many strains, but a cold was a cold. Hepatitis B was serious. Eventually, our cases were deemed to be hepatitis B, but we still wondered which of the combination of factors we faced truly caused us to get it.

Strangely, as word spread around that our little group had been afflicted with "B"; we became more popular than ever. I suppose that had to do with the usual anti-authority rebellion students of the time were immersed within, because the adults at school and some at home considered us nothing short of evil. In their eyes, we had broken the rules and God was punishing us for that, pure and simple.

Regardless of what we believed about the causes, the "punishment" part was highly evident as our disease progressed. The utter weakness and fatigue that overcomes the body when hepatitis is present sometimes became so unbearable that my very will to live was challenged. My appetite was almost non-existent during the peak of the disease, and so was my energy level.

Friends would call and say, "let's go" when it was time for swimming or surfing, and I tried to get away with telling them I just didn't feel like it. They'd show up anyway, hoping to convince me to get off my butt and come along, but when they saw the skinny, yellow, despondent boy I had become, they would give up and go ahead without me.

That was punishment, too.

Fortunately, with my class hovering at around 950 students, there were plenty of other scandals to distract attention away from the group of us that had hepatitis-B. By the time we were seniors, the effects of the disease had gone away and we could attend school more regularly, but not without the memories of the yellow mark that jaundice had painted on our faces.

To many of our peers, we had become celebrities. At graduation, our yearbooks were signed with things like *"Dear Mello Yellow,"* or *"You All Live in the Yellow Submarine."* As I watched those words being scribbled on the pages, I did my best to be a man and hold back the tears. I knew my classmates weren't trying to hurt me, but they couldn't hope to understand the profound impact my disease had made on me.

More punishment...

When I got home from our graduation ceremony, I took one last glance at one of the more wicked entries someone had made:

"Yellow Haze, all in my brain. . .
Excuse me, while I miss the sky"

I was tired of missing the sky. I threw that yearbook away right then, unable to hold back the tears any longer. I may have been on the threshold of manhood, but I could not be expected to be a man right now.

Not even if I was bulletproof.

Another Statistic

Faced with the news that my liver was for all practical purposes 96% *gone*, I turned my attention to the wonderful array of options I now had for doing something about it.

By now, I had shelved the idea of seeking a second opinion. It seemed fruitless, really, and a genuine waste of what little time I might have left. Instead, I would consider what I had been told by the Doc at Mississippi University Medical, and try to make some sense of the mess my life was fast becoming.

For her part, the director of Gastroenterology had advised immediate steps to get me placed on the liver donor's waiting list; time to drop a new one in and erase all the damage that my "Non A-non B" case of hepatitis had wrought.

The realities of preparing for a major operation like a liver transplant are not very uplifting. Before giving me one of the 5,000[5] or so livers that wind up with new owners each year, the doctors would want to know that I'd be a worthy recipient.

There would be tests--lots of tests.

First, they would evaluate the rest of my physical condition. They would want to know that my heart wasn't facing imminent failure from lack of exercise, poor diet or previous damage from progressive heart disease. They would perform EKG's, stress tests, and blood gas evaluations.

How about those lungs? Had I set myself up for lung cancer by smoking tobacco? Was I going to suffer respiratory consequences either from my behaviors or from the rigors of the liver transplant?

---

[5] http://www.organdonor.gov/student/access/organs.asp

Stomach, intestines, and colon would also have to be examined. They would insert camera tubes down my throat and into my stomach; the same for the other end. If they found enlarged veins (called varicies) present in my digestive system, they would tie them off with rubber bands to prevent them from bleeding.

They would order MRI's, CAT scans, and X-rays. There would be all manner of needles poking me to take blood samples, and abundant tests for previous diseases like tuberculosis and more ordinary infections.

In addition to the microscope my physical body would be placed beneath, the doctors would want to scrutinize my mental health as well. How well does he handle stress? Does he have a supportive family? Will he call the whole thing off 10 minutes before the anesthesiologist shows up?

There would be dieticians called in to investigate my nutritional needs and habits. While I had done my best to follow a good nutritional plan since being told I had hepatitis again back in 1983, there was little doubt these dieticians would have ideas of their own.

When all of these tests and reports and observations were "done," the results would be presented to a transplant committee for review. This committee would try to satisfy itself that I wouldn't waste my new liver either by inconveniently dying of something else or jumping off a bridge. And if they managed to do that, the committee would bestow upon me the honor of a place on their precious liver waiting list, where I would become one of 17,000[6] or so people competing for one of those 5,000 livers someone else was unlucky enough to donate.

Like I said, not very uplifting.

The irony of the situation doesn't end with the long odds of even *getting* a new liver, either. As I began to educate myself about the realities of going through a liver transplant, I remembered the University Medical doctor's proud declaration that almost 75% of liver donor recipients survive for five years after the transplant.

So let me get this straight.

---

[6] http://www.organdonor.gov/student/access/organs.asp

I'm supposed to go through all of this trauma, this pain and this suffering and shock and distress and this *ordeal*, just so I *might* survive for five more years? And what about *after* five years? How many patients make it six, seven, ten or twenty years?

"None," she had said bluntly. "We express the outlook for liver transplant patients as a five-year survival rate."[7]

Thinking about that grim eventuality, I was finding it hard to get on board with the whole "let's find Johnny a new liver" thing. To me, saying yes to the long journey required just to get a spot on the liver waiting list was saying yes to give up.

While I could no longer deny that I was dying, I didn't think that I had to give up. Praying on it hard in the hours following the University Medical Doc's blunt declarations, I decided I would tell her just that.

I decided that Johnny Delirious would not be asking for a new liver after all.

---

[7] http://www.liverfoundation.org/education/info/transplant/

The Establishment

With high school behind me and my parents doing their best to nudge along my decisions about the future, the climate in 1971 was nothing short of chaotic.

In the days following my graduation, 36 people were hospitalized after drinking LSD-spiked apple juice at a Grateful Dead concert. President Nixon had ordered the arrests of over 10,000 anti-war protestors, and there were the riots at Attica, as well as Brooklyn, Chattanooga, and even closer to home in Jacksonville.[8]

During this tumultuous time, there was still room for growth. The state of Washington became the first to ban sex discrimination. Voting rights were granted to us 18-year olds. Federal Express, Greenpeace, National Public Radio, Amtrak and the NASDAQ were all born. The cost of a postage stamp went up 33% (to eight cents) for a first-class letter.[9]

My father's medical practice grew during this time as well. He was a fixture at the clinic where he worked, and fully ensconced within what we teenagers were now calling the "The Establishment."

To us, "The Establishment" went beyond the industrial-military complex and really, it could mean just about anything that was accepted as a social "norm." It was the time of Malcolm X and Dr. Martin Luther King, Jr. And it was a time of great turbulence in our country.

While during this time I became less involved with my church, I still believed in Jesus. Many of us who were "anti-establishment" didn't struggle with any sense of being "anti-Jesus" just because we

---

[8] http://www.brainyhistory.com/years/1971.html
[9] http://www.thepeoplehistory.com/1971.html

didn't agree with all things "normal." In fact, there were some who made a strong case that Jesus himself was "anti-establishment," because he went against the wishes of those in power during his time.

My own skirmishes with The Establishment began at home. In my eyes, my father was The Establishment personified. In the early 1970's, I remember watching *All in the Family*, better known as the "Archie Bunker Show" with my dad quite often. It was one of our favorite shows, albeit for different reasons.

My dad identified quite readily with Archie, who in the show was as "Establishment" as you could get. Archie's character perfectly represented the thoughts and sensibilities of people within my dad's ilk who really didn't like the idea of change. They were set in their ways, old-fashioned to be sure, and not at all embracing the more modern, open-minded thinking we teenagers were practicing.

When I watched *All in the Family*, I related to "Meathead," Archie's liberal son-in-law. My dad was all about Archie. He not only related to the character that Carol O'Conner played; there were times when he downright *agreed* with the thoughts and ideas that Archie portrayed. Funny to think that when we both laughed out loud at Archie's pontifications, one of us was laughing because he was shocked, the other because he approved.

All in the Family captured an Emmy in 1971 for its ability to create that kind of paradox. Indeed, the early '70's were themselves a paradox among us who went to junior college, with big social divisions between jocks, burnouts, preppies, cheerleaders, and the "hip" crowd. Above all, we were divided most clearly by those who went to Vietnam and those who didn't.

According to a Harris poll taken at the time, 60% of the American people were becoming "Anti Establishment" through their disapproval of the Vietnam War.[10] Equal restlessness existed about the draft, as many young men of my age wrestled with the decision to burn their draft cards, have kids, or outright flee the country for the safer surroundings in Canada.

For me, dodging the draft and my duty along with it was never something I seriously considered. I did, however, have a plan in place to address the situation should I find myself with a draft number that was low enough to put me in danger of being forcibly enlisted. I

---

[10] http://www.thepeoplehistory.com/1971.html

figured that rather than waiting for the call from the Army, I'd simply sign up voluntarily for the Air Force. This way, I would at least be able to designate my career choice instead of letting the military choose the infantry for me. And since I liked to work in the kitchen, I would apply to become an Air Force cook, giving me a chance to contribute to the effort without having to kill anybody in the process. Fortunately for me, things never came even close to that.

When I got my draft card in 1971, the number at the top read "343 H." Since the highest number you could get was 365, this meant that the likelihood of me being drafted was very low. I could only be called to report after the men who had drawn the numbers 1 through 342, and since I had an "H" labeling me as a "Hold" my chances were even better. "Holds" would not be called before those who had an "A" designating them as immediately ready to report.

So I was lucky, a fact that my friends were eager to remind me of every chance they got. Some of those friends, however, were not so blessed. Some of them went to Vietnam. And some of them did not come back. Some of the ones that did told me stories that made me shudder. Not just because of the garden variety horrors of war, but also because of some of the secret things the military was doing.

There were entire livelihoods and careers made by some military men, a result of the importation of illegal substances from Vietnam. There were military men who died in the usual ways that war will bring. There were those who died even after they arrived "safely" home, unable to cope with the conviction that they were patriotic while hearing the roar of the crowd that screamed they weren't. Some died, both abroad and at home, of diseases that were no longer even thought about in the United States.

There were even some that died of hepatitis.

Acceptance

Just about everyone in my life was furious with me. The docs at University Medical. My sisters. My brother. My Friends.
Everybody.
None of them could understand my decision to forego a liver transplant. All of them were sure it was going to be the decision that did me in, once and for all, such that I would be taking the Dirt Nap some time within the next eight months.

In truth, by now I had accepted my situation far more completely than my family had. Don't get me wrong – I had not accepted my doctors' assertions that saying "no" to a new liver meant saying "yes" to death. Rather, I had accepted the fact that my liver wasn't going to do its job in its present state. And I accepted the responsibility of trying to find a way to survive nonetheless.

This was a responsibility that I knew I could not take lightly. Nor would it be easy. But I was certainly not ready to give up, and I was far from ready for drug cocktails and clinical tests that would dominate my every waking moment.

I wasn't ready to sit around and wait for someone else with a healthy liver to die, either.

Determined to prove the doctors and my family wrong, I decided to trade the operating table for a more natural path to getting myself healed. This was not an easy decision; I was scared and unsure and it was hard to ignore the voices of the people in my life who were telling me I was crazy.

But signing up for a liver transplant that only might be successful, just so that I might survive for five years after the surgery?

Now *that* was crazy.

Mexico, Squared

By 1974, my experiences at "Hepatitis High" were a distant memory. As a result, I was able to focus on some of my more artistic abilities, and I got into making feather jewelry. The feather "chokers" and earrings that I made for women, along with the cowboy hats for the men, were in enough demand to allow me to sell a fair amount of the stuff. In turn, I was able to make a reasonable living.

I also got into restoring old cars during this time. For me, this was truly a craft, and I got a real kick out of the attention my work received when I went to art shows. But expenses incurred while I attended some of those shows were high enough that they often exceeded my profits. As I contemplated my next steps, I turned my thoughts to a new adventure where I could make the modest dollars I earned last a bit longer.

Thus, Mexico came to mind.

In the mid 1970's, the dollar had nearly three times the buying power in Mexico that it did in the U.S. For a young, Anti-Establishment type like me, that was a pretty alluring difference. Accordingly, I came to see living in Mexico as a chance to make my money stretch a little, learn another language, and expand my horizons with a bit of worldliness to boot.

The decision to establish new roots in Mexico had nothing to do with a lack of love for my country. Anti-Establishment or not, I was an American, albeit one that was getting a little weary of the direction some of the social scenes were taking at home. Weary and disillusioned, sort of like Robert in Hemmingway's *For Whom The Bell Tolls*.

Not wanting to get caught any deeper in the wrong holes, I decided to go for it and enrolled at the University of the Americas in Puebla, Mexico.

Puebla is situated 110 km southeast of Mexico City in a valley that is surrounded by volcanoes and mountains. The snow-capped volcanoes jutting upward in the distance are glorious to behold at any time of the year. At 7,000 feet above sea level, the city's climate is cooler in winter and moderate in summer, making it more tolerable than the blistering heat much of Mexico is famous for.[11]

Puebla is something of a mini-melting pot, with a history of immigration from Europe in the late 1800's to early 1900's. There are Italian and German influences, quite to the point that one section of the city hosts a full-blown *Oktoberfest* in the fall.[12] The city also hosts more than 20 universities,[13] and the one I chose was perennially ranked near the top in all of Mexico.

My time at the University of the Americas would prove to be every bit as enlightening as I had hoped it would. Through most of 1974 and 1975, I studied primarily Spanish Literature and both colonial and pre-Columbian Latin American history. These were satisfying courses for me, but as an art lover, my ears perked up when other students told me about San Miguel de Allende and the art institute there.

Located about 170 miles from Mexico City, the *Instituto Allende* was fast becoming a hot-spot for writers, artists and musicians from all over the world. There were a lot of American students there, too, so I had the luxury of mixing with the locals without losing the ability to stay in touch with what was going on at home. I found it to be a highly stimulating place to spend time, as it was abundant with true artists who were steadfastly committed to their various disciplines.

Being around people like that made me feel like I had finally arrived. I made it official when I enrolled at the *Instituto*, and although I wasn't painting and sculpting like a modern Leonardo Da Vinci, I felt I had found my place with my coursework and my study.

---

[11] http://en.wikipedia.org/wiki/Puebla,_Puebla
[12] http://en.wikipedia.org/wiki/Puebla,_Puebla
[13] http://en.wikipedia.org/wiki/Puebla,_Puebla

The experience at the *Instituto Allende* served to magnify my interest and my skill when it came to feather jewelry. I had made the assembly of the jewelry my primary trade while I was in Mexico, but I also managed to get a bit of leverage from my beach-boy days in Florida. Taking advantage of my abilities as a strong swimmer, I worked the weekends as a lifeguard at one of the many local resorts. Between that and my jewelry business, I was doing well enough to pay my way through a true life's experience that I would always hold as one of my finest.

--

Toward the middle of 1976, I decided to head back to the U.S. for a spell and use my newly honed artistic skills to take advantage of the turquoise jewelry craze of the time. Selling the jewelry at one of the most popular seafood restaurants near Fort Walton Beach, I managed to squeeze out some marginal profits. In an effort to expand my reach, I later went into business with a jewelry store and a boutique. All good fun, but unfortunately the retail world was never going to make me independently wealthy, even after three years of earnest hard work at it. Just as my father had predicted, the turquoise jewelry fad was short-lived, "here today, gone tomorrow," kind of like the Hula Hoop.

Feeling a little disheartened by the whole series of events, my thoughts turned once again to Mexico and the time I had enjoyed in San Miguel de Allende. With little to lose and no heavy anchors to keep me at home, in 1980 I decided to head back down south of the border and pick up where I left off in Mexico.

--

My second foray into the world of *Tierra Azteca* brought me close to another kind of art form that was different from those I had studied thus far; different, but certainly more rewarding.

When you think of Kung Fu, you probably don't think of Mexico. And sure enough, it wasn't a native of my second country that got me into this fascinating new form of expression. Instead, it was a martial arts master from San Francisco. His name was Peter.

At least six evenings every week, Peter tutored me in Kung Fu, in much the same way as David Carradine from the TV show. I was Peter's "Grasshopper," and I could not help but think of myself as Carradine while we worked out, marking the hours as the church bells rang a few blocks away from our spot on an *Instituto* porch overlooking the historic old town. The memories of those evening hours would spill into my mind for many years to come, the same way the shadows crept across the old buildings of San Miguel as we worked to sharpen our craft.

Though my skills in Kung Fu had become honed to a respectable level, they could not protect me from enemies I couldn't see. My second stint in Mexico required that I return to the States once per year to renew my visa, and on one of those trips northward I met up with an old nemesis in a most unfortunate way.

In 1983, stopping for a bite to eat before crossing the border back into the U.S., I made the fateful decision to try a shrimp cocktail. It didn't taste badly at all, though the shrimp was drenched with hot sauce, so if it wasn't fresh or if it was tainted I probably wouldn't have been able to tell.

My liver, on the other hand, revealed the quality of the shellfish quite noticeably the next day. I was yellow from head to toe with jaundice, and I knew right away that I was sick again.

Hepatitis High, Mexico style.

When I got back to the states, I headed to Jackson, MS to stay with my brother for a few days with the hope of recuperating quickly. When the mirror showed me my yellow face each morning in the days that followed, I finally relented and went to University Medical in Jackson to have some testing done. When the results came back, they showed I did indeed have hepatitis again. This time, though, it wasn't just "A" or "B." It was a new strain they were calling "Non A, non-B" hepatitis.

Wonderful, I thought, this is a whole new way to experience the magnificent world of liver disease.

Without much else to offer in the way of treatment options, the doctors suggested I continue with a healthy eating regimen, avoid alcohol, caffeine, and pretty much any other liquid except purified water, and return to my brother's house for some serious rest.

So rest I did. At meal times, I gorged myself on copious quantities of fruit and red beans and rice. I adhered to the rest of the doctor's orders, and somehow after a few weeks I was myself again.

No more *Mello Yellow.*

--

With a fresh visa and my liver on the mend, I returned to San Miguel to continue my studies in the arts. By now, Peter had become my best friend, and some evenings we worked the barrio haunts together for studies of a different kind.

The women of Mexico can be as enchanting as any I'd ever met in Florida. I had my share of flings with the local girls and would not have hesitated to pursue a serious relationship with the right one, but it turns out my two most meaningful connections wound up being with women who were students at the *Instituto,* just like me. Neither of them were from Mexico, or anywhere else in North America, for that matter.

Meeting people from different countries and cultures was not at all unusual in San Miguel, since the *Instituto* is a world-renowned place to study. While most of the foreign students came from the United States, it wasn't out of the ordinary to meet students that hailed from Europe. Thus, when I fell in love with a girl from France, it was no more unexpected than if I had gotten serious with an American or Mexican gal. And although there weren't many Asians attending at the *Instituto,* as luck would have it another of the most memorable relationships in my lifetime wound up being with a girl from Japan.

Dating each girl over a period of six years (yes, there was a one-year gap; I was never a "juggler" that stayed in more than one relationship at a time) things would get serious enough that we talked of marriage in both cases. Talked in Spanish, that is, since neither girl spoke English.

I visited each girl's parents in their home countries, making the trip to Nice in France and Tokyo in Japan. Both sets of parents accepted and liked me enough to grant me their daughters' hand in matrimony. Both families were wealthy enough to eliminate worry about finances, too. The French girl's parents were fourth-generation vintners, and they were actually gracious enough to pay for my round-trip airfare when we visited them in France.

On those two occasions, the relationships were deep enough that I might have settled down and gotten married. But in both cases, I felt that my love wasn't as strong as theirs, and with the scales tipped too far one way I couldn't let things go on. I broke off both relationships eventually, and both girls went on to forge great careers and great lives for themselves, particularly the one from Japan. She took what she learned about Mexican cuisine in San Miguel back to Tokyo, where she started the first chain of Mexican restaurants in Japan. She was later recognized nationally as an exceptional female entrepreneur, no small feat in the male-dominated business world of Japan.

It felt good to see both of the girls succeed, almost as if it reinforced my instincts about their good character. On the other hand, it felt a bit sad not to be a part of their success longer than I was, but I knew that I had made the right decision in each case just the same. I always did my best to avoid being deceitful when it came to matters of the heart.

In the years to follow, though, I would come to wish that my body would afford me the same courtesy regarding matters of the liver.

Going Natural

Throwing conventional medicine to the wind in favor of a more natural approach to curing my hepatitis was not an easy thing to do by any means. I had been no stranger to healthy eating in the years since my 1983 diagnosis of what would soon become known as hepatitis "C," but now I had to ask myself if I could repair 96% of my damaged liver simply by eating right.

Even though I was doing my best to ignore the naysayers, which included just about everyone I had ever met, there were times when I got scared and gave fleeting thought to reconsidering the doctors' pleas to get me going on drug cocktails and interferon. But I was steadfast in my opposition to a liver transplant, because I simply saw it as a sure way to find myself dead in five years. By going natural instead, I could leave my situation in my own hands and if things didn't work out, at the very least I could ensure that I'd go out happy and content instead of miserably wasting away in hospitals for the rest of my days.

Yes, I was scared. Make no mistake about it. But I knew that my health and my well being were heavily dependent upon an affirmative frame of mind, so I threw away the foreboding pessimism and replaced it with intense concentration on finding alternative, natural treatments for my condition. Such focus not only occupied my mind and kept me from going whacko, but it also provided me with some hope in the form of something therapeutic from the health food store to take.

Milk thistle.

With a long stem and spiky leaves, this ugly-looking flowering plant would easily be dismissed as an ordinary weed by most people. But my research showed that for over 2,000 years, the extract from milk thistle seeds has been used in medicine to treat disorders of the digestive system, including those of the liver.[14]

The active ingredient in milk thistle is silymarin, and with doses of 230-600 mg per day, adults over 18 with chronic hepatitis have shown improved liver tests in some studies[15]. Of course, the doomsday theorists in my life would point to the negative data, saying that the studies done to date were "inconclusive" or had been poorly engineered. True, there were disclaimers about side effects and the overall usefulness of silymarin, including this one from the Mayo Clinic:

"The U.S. Food and Drug Administration does not strictly regulate herbs and supplements. There is no guarantee of strength, purity, or safety of products, and effects may vary."[16]

But for a man grasping at straws, the thorny stalk of the milk thistle plant was looking like something I should clutch as ferverently as the hope for recovery I was holding onto. To me, it seemed obvious that at this stage I should focus on the optimistic nature of the reports from Europe that were out there, and thus I dove in and took the maximum recommended dose every day.

Along with the milk thistle extract, I drank teas made from mint and dandelions. Dandelion tea, much like milk thistle, has been used for centuries as a natural remedy for afflictions of the kidneys and the liver.[17] So between the silymarin and the dandelion tea, I was getting my fill of weeds that were a bit less hallucinogenic than the ones I had puffed upon in my younger days.

The rest of my diet would be very clean and very simple; more red beans and brown rice, plenty of watermelon, oatmeal and vitamin-C rich oranges and no meat or animal products.

This was the beginning of my plan for a natural start to heal myself. If I could make it work just well enough to regain some of my faded strength, then I could get serious about pouring all of my energy into a holistic recovery. So, armed with some new-found confidence

---

[14] http://www.mayoclinic.com/health/silymarin/NS_patient-milkthistle
[15] http://www.mayoclinic.com/health/silymarin/NS_patient-milkthistle
[16] http://www.mayoclinic.com/health/silymarin/NS_patient-milkthistle
[17] http://www.dandeliontea.org/

in having a better strategy for survival than the one my doctors gave me, I settled in for some much-needed relaxation and plenty of sleep.

Rest, after all, is a magnificent weapon.

Laboratory Life

My incredible experiences in San Miguel behind me, I came back to the U.S. for good in 1985. During that year, Ronald Reagan was sworn in for a second term, Coca-Cola tried to change its long-successful recipe, UK scientists foretold global warming with the announcement of a large hole in the ozone layer, and Rock Hudson became the first major U.S. entertainer to die of AIDS.[18]

With unemployment hovering around 7% and interest rates still struggling to get below double-digits, Americans were getting worried about government spending approaching one trillion dollars in a single year.[19]

Besides the state of affairs within the economy, Americans were also as worried as ever about their health. New and promising treatments and techniques throughout the world of medicine were getting a lot of attention, and with my own dubious medical history they got my attention, too.

One advancement that showed a lot of potential was the continued development of hair analysis technology. Hair analysis had first come on the scene in the 1970's, and advocates of the procedure considered it useful for identifying the overall condition of a person's state of health. The process consists of elemental analysis of a hair follicle from the subject in question, with the intention of spotting toxins that are detrimental to the subject's well being.[20] It has been used as a preferred method for forensic study and drug testing, and although the validity of the technique has been questioned in some circles, I was intrigued by the idea. To my way of thinking, it is hard

---

[18] http://www.infoplease.com/year/1985.html
[19] http://www.infoplease.com/year/1985.html
[20] http://www.hairanalysisprogram.com/what-is-a-hair-analysis.php

to name a revolutionary development of any kind that doesn't have its detractors.

So in 1985 when I heard about a hair analysis laboratory for sale in Dallas, my ears perked up. With a tentative inquiry, I found out that for a small investment I could own the company and become an entrepreneur again, hopefully with a longer record of success than my jewelry business had afforded me in the past.

The founder of the Dallas company was a man by the name of Jim Davenport. Jim was a true pioneer who had put the science of hair analysis itself on the map, treating the determination of heavy metal toxicity in the hair as a valuable source of information that should be utilized more readily within the medical community.

After meeting Jim and finding out a bit more about hair analysis, I took a leap of faith and invested in the business, and in return, Jim stayed on to educate me about the field. In addition to Davenport's expertise, we had Jeffrey Bland as the company's Director. Bland was one of the top organic chemists in the country, so his background represented a big contribution to the viability of our business.

Learning from Davenport and Bland was a privilege to me. They were both very knowledgeable and they taught me a lot about the value of hair analysis and what it could mean to medical diagnostics. The elemental reports that came back from our hair analysis testing revealed a host of information that could be indispensable when evaluating numerous key health-related factors. I would come to learn that hair analysis is effective in determining a wide variety of conditions, including the following:

- Levels of toxic elements, which can be indicators of pathological disorders[21]
- Levels of elements crucial to good health that are present in the body[22]
- Vitamin deficiencies[23]
- Various nutritional deficiencies[24]

---

[21] http://www.hairanalysisprogram.com/what-is-a-hair-analysis.php
[22] http://www.hairanalysisprogram.com/what-is-a-hair-analysis.php
[23] http://www.hairanalysistest.com/
[24] http://www.hairanalysistest.com/

Some proponents of hair analysis contend that the hair tissue is affected by many factors, including environmental issues, genetics, hormones, and enzymes.[25] As such, the practice of hair analysis can be a window that shows through to what is being stored in the body, and thus it can be useful for diagnostics and even recommended treatment paths.

Of course, Davenport Labs was not the only firm on the planet that saw the value in hair analysis. By the mid 1980's, competition designed to take advantage of the benefits of the process was not exactly in short supply. And some of those competitors were adopting automated testing methods that were putting a major squeeze on the ability to turn a profit at this new game. Our own company had a solid customer base consisting of medical doctors and heath care practitioners, but as cost and expenses grew, the only way to expand the business was to climb aboard the automated testing bandwagon.

So much for a "small" investment.

It didn't take long to determine that buying or leasing automated equipment would drive our monthly expenses to a level beyond our expected income. So, faced with the choice of "growing" into a long-term bankruptcy or maintaining the business with our conventional testing methods, I chose the latter. This choice meant that I could only defer the inevitable, because larger firms with deeper pockets could use their modernized facilities to provide testing cheaper than we could. Predictably, this led to the thinning of our customer base, despite our contention that Davenport's testing methods were more accurate than the automated ones.

My second foray into the world of business ownership took just as sharp a toll on me as my first. I found myself getting fatigued earlier and earlier in the day, until I finally succumbed to the stress and pressure to the point of sleeping late on work days. More and more, my productivity, my mood and my energy levels all went down.

It seemed that the business was getting worse and I was getting worse. In fact, blood tests would later confirm that my hepatitis C was flaring up again. I was not feeling good, it was impossible for me to finance an expansion of my business, and I was finding it harder and harder to remain immersed in the declining circumstances I was once again experiencing.

---

[25] http://www.hairanalysistest.com/

I was forced to make some hard decisions, and so I did. I sold the assets of Davenport Labs, making my official record as a business tycoon zero for two.

War

If rest can be considered a weapon to use in battle, then exercise must be viewed as an army to be deployed in war. To be sure, I was indeed fighting a war and no amount of rest would be enough to help me overcome my disease.

I could not shake the thought that my state of mind was absolutely crucial to my quest for a natural cure. And for me, there were two things essential to the very core of my mental well-being:

*Exercising my mind through
the pursuit of knowledge*

*Exercising my body through
the pursuit of peak physical condition*

For these reasons, I decided it was time to leave my brother's house in Mississippi and head home to Florida, where I could accelerate my chase for optimum mental and physical fitness. Realistically, I didn't need to be close to the University Medical center anymore, because I wasn't listening to their ideas about how to get "better" anyway. And I had finished my studies at Hinds Junior College in Jackson with honors, so maybe it was time again for the challenge of higher learning like I had experienced in Mexico.

Pensacola, therefore, would be my next stop. It was essentially home to me, being only 40 miles away from Fort Walton Beach, and just now home sounded pretty good. I figured that if I was going to die in another seven months or so, I might as well die at home and I might as well die as smart and physically fit as I could be.

Besides, fat guys look silly when they're stuffed into a casket; it makes the pallbearers all sweaty, too.

By now, I had enough of my strength back to make the trek to Florida and set up a new place to hang my hat, but my test results were really no better. Everyone was still wagering that I was not long for this world. Nevertheless, I was going to do my best to make them all lose that bet. Thus, there was simply no need to stick around and face more gloomy medical news, all of which would serve only to fly in the face of my plans for superior emotional healthiness.

Signing up for junior-level classes at the University of Western Florida, I stated my major as communications, with emphasis on marketing, journalism and politics. For such a degree I would need computer courses as well, which afforded me the opportunity to get maximum use of the Internet for researching holistic methods of stabilizing my hepatitis C. In fact, I lost myself completely for many hours at a time in front of those computer screens, my ravenous appetite for healing knowledge becoming nothing short of a deep obsession.

As for the physical part of my conditioning, I could think of no better strategy than to turn back to my passion for Kung Fu. My buddy Peter was still living in San Miguel, so he wasn't going to be able to serve as my teacher. Fortunately for me, however, I met a true master right there in Pensacola. This one happened to be from Iran, which is no surprise since Kung Fu has a storied history in what used to be Persia. Quite apparently, the masters from the Middle East are every bit as sharp as any from India or China, and my teacher was no exception.

One difference between my new teacher and Peter back in Mexico was the utter fierceness with which he approached Kung Fu. The practice routines were insanely rigorous, and I guess they had to be, because many of my fellow students were absolute, unqualified *badasses* in every way. Even most of the women who trained with us males were hellions in their own right. True, they didn't stack up completely with the Navy Seals or SWAT-team students in our group, but they were potent and aggressive just the same. Many of these women had taken up martial arts to protect themselves against repeating the experience of being abused or raped. And they were very proficient at trading their fear for the more proactive choice of using lightning-fast kicks and punches.

My purpose in re-joining the pursuit of excellence in Kung Fu had nothing to do with the desire to be a badass myself. Rather, I saw it as a way to step up the effort to beat my disease. Reflecting back upon my time with Peter at the *Instituto*, I remembered thinking of myself as David Carradine in the TV show *Kung Fu*. And now, with my liver disease progressing to the point of near catastrophe, I found myself identifying with that character even more profoundly.

In one particular episode of the show, I remembered Carradine's Master healing him when he was critically ill. It was a flashback scene for Carradine's character, just like my ruminations about Peter and my early training in Kung Fu were now. In Carradine's version, he was remembering his Master's ability to heal, and in the show he applied what he learned to the benefit of a sick native-American. His patient was cured through the strength of Carradine's faith in the practices taught to him by his Master, such that the Grasshopper had become a Master himself.

In all the years since I had seen that episode, I could never manage to push it out of my mind. If strict adherence to the study of Kung Fu could help Carradine's character to be a healer in the show, then why couldn't it help me?

Was it really possible for Grasshopper to win a war?

Well, I supposed that without reinforcements in the form of liver transplants or drug concoctions, I was going to find out soon enough.

The Zapper

Frank Zappa and Audrey Hepburn died, as I recall, right around the same time I started even more intensive research about alternative therapies for my hepatitis C.

My work was downright exhaustive, encompassing everything I could find out regarding natural health, therapies and herbs. I studied the shelves of the health food store and I studied countless pages of the worldwide web. Inevitably, I found plenty of ideas that would best be described as outright quackery, but to be fair, perhaps the more orbital concepts out there had helped *someone*.

Take Dr. Hulda Clark, for example. Clark is the innovator behind a controversial method of scanning the human body electronically for the purpose of uncovering the presence of certain diseases. One of her central theories revolves around the idea that cancer is caused by parasites in the body. In addition to the conventional definition of "parasites," which to most people covers things like tapeworms, flukes and roundworms, Dr. Clark employs an expanded view. She includes bacteria, fungi, molds and viruses as part of the parasite family.[26] And she firmly believes that killing unwanted parasites in the body is one of the keys to restoring good, natural health in people who have all manner of terminal diseases.

Some of Hulda's critics have considered her non-mainstream ideas as "out there," going so far as to call her claims "bizarre." She has had to face litigation as well. I saw from my evaluation of the benefits of milk thistle and hair analysis, and recalling my curriculum in grade school; that history has taught us that revolutionaries are often labeled as crackpots (or worse). After all, the ideas of people like

---

[26] http://www.drclark.ch/en/products_devices/devices/zapper.php

Christopher Columbus and Galileo were not only considered absurd in their time, but in many cases contrarian thinking was enough to get a person burned alive at the stake.

As such, I dismissed Dr. Clark's attackers and read up on her methods and techniques. And lacking a whole bunch of alternatives that didn't involve tearing out what was left of my liver; I decided to give one of Dr. Clark's approaches a shot.

Enter the Zapper.

For less than $100, I engaged the services of a local freelance electrician, and I had him duplicate Dr. Clark's "Zapper" device from the schematics she included in her book, *The Cure for all Diseases*. The Zapper is used to literally electrocute parasites, bacteria and viruses of all kinds,[27] without causing damage to vital bodily tissues.[28]

I followed Dr. Clark's instructions for using the device, summarily pumping alternating current into my flesh at 30,000 cycles per second. The selection of such a high electrical frequency was made so that Dr. Clark could maximize the *current* flow to the affected areas, yet leave the voltage very low, such that side effects and any physical harm are not significant concerns. The thing operates on just a 9-volt battery for that very reason.[29]

Using the process regularly as advised by Dr. Clark, I believed that the Zapper did indeed help my body to rid itself of many of the things that could be contributing to the ugly state of affairs with my liver. I had no proof of this. I had no extensive medical testing done that would show the difference between the presence of things like fluke worms both before and after the Zapper treatments.

But I believed it helped, and even if I couldn't prove the extent to which the Zapper was contributing, the very fact that *I believed it helped* may have been just as therapeutic as anything the device itself could deliver.

Dr. Clark's research and subsequent writing served to firmly reinforce my commitment to a natural cure for my disease. Besides her advocacy of using electrical means to rid the body of parasites, she was a strong supporter of herbal therapy as well. Her study at the Clayton College of Natural Health led to her degree in Naturopathy, and seeing a person of her credentials emphasize the importance of

---

[27] http://www.relfe.com/hulda_clark.html
[28] http://www.drclark.ch/en/products_devices/devices/zapper.php
[29] http://www.drclark.ch/en/products_devices/devices/zapper.php

staying on the very path of natural, herbal treatment I was pursuing was therapeutic for me, too.

--

Attending Alcoholics Anonymous meetings was never something I thought I would need in my younger days. Never one to drink abusively, I had merely engaged in the same sort of social imbibing that friends and relatives typically enjoyed whenever the occasion seemed appropriate. Yes, like most human beings, I had my share of mild binges that led to the occasional heavy "buzz," but I had never been pulled over for driving drunk and I certainly never "needed" alcohol to get myself through the day.

Nevertheless, to a hepatitis C sufferer, alcohol of any kind is Kryptonite, pure and simple. Especially in my case, with only 4% of my liver surviving scar-tissue free, it was critical to my well-being to avoid even an innocent glass of wine as a compliment to a fine meal. For me, the fact that I was not a heavy alcohol user notwithstanding, it was still hard to forego the satisfying taste of a cold, crisp beer in the steamy afternoons of Florida's oppressive summer heat.

Hence my enrollment with the Pensacola chapter of AA.

The Alcoholics Anonymous meetings were a therapy of their own kind, and they facilitated in me a mindset that would later prove useful when I became involved in support groups for people with terminal diseases. They also facilitated my ability to swear off alcohol entirely, a development that I considered critical to any hope for a meaningful recovery.

I would miss that blissful glass of red wine and that throat-burning, thirst-quenching bottle of beer. But clean and sober I was, and I would remain dedicated to staying that way however long I might have left to live.

--

Being back home in Florida for more than a semester now, I had my share of class papers to toil over in my studies at the University of Western Florida. I usually got pretty good grades, but I found my best marks came when I worked extra hard to provide something that my classmates might find helpful, especially when it was a well-researched paper with good sources cited along the way.

Living in a one-bedroom apartment close to the campus, it was easy for me to walk back and forth between classes and home. And home was close to the local Mecca for us health-food enthusiasts, in the form of Everman's Natural Foods Co-Op in Pensacola.

Everman's status as a Co-Op meant that it was a collection of local people with common interests and goals, among them being the pursuit of wellness through adopting a healthy-eating lifestyle. The Co-Op standing of the store also meant that successful operation required volunteers for everything from stocking shelves to teaching cooking classes. With a vested interest in the sustainability of the Co-Op, I signed up to volunteer and over time, I became known as a bit of a fixture at Everman's. Eventually, a few of the patrons would come to regard me as something of a celebrity, too.

The sense of belongingness and purpose I obtained through my efforts at the Co-Op were building blocks to the overall reconstruction of my psychological vitality. When I was at my best my confidence soared, and I allowed myself to believe maybe I really would find a way to Zap this hep-C thing right on out of my liver, once and for all.

Peace

Death, for all of its drawbacks, would at least offer a kind of peace, wouldn't it?

Plunging with unabashed faith into the world of natural treatments and holistic therapies was redeeming in so many ways, but it was also terrifying at the same time. Some days, it was kind of like accelerating toward a brick wall in the car you were borrowing for driver's education, your teacher screaming in the seat beside you to *HIT THE BRAKES!* Consumed with the desire for self-preservation, he keeps slamming his foot into the floorboard in an effort to save you from yourself, except he doesn't have one of those fancy, "time out for safety" dual-brake systems so he can't stop the car. Only you can.

But you don't. You just keep tearing along, the pedal all the way maxed to the floor, the needle on the tach stretching way past the redline and the wall getting bigger and bigger in the windshield all the time.

It's a hellish game of chicken, really.

Playing "chicken" with my life was never something that was very high on my "things to do before I die" list. But there were days I felt that was exactly what I was doing.

There were people way smarter than me telling me so. They were telling me every chance they got, in no uncertain terms and without an ounce of compassion or understanding.

When they did that to me, it was hard to ignore a lot of what they were spewing. Evidence, they would say, points strongly in the opposite direction you are heading.

Take the medicines!
Drink the drug cocktails!

Shop around a little and pick yourself up a shiny, brand new liver!

But I hung tough, refusing to trade one kind of death for another. When I had momentary lapses in confidence, I would paint a picture of myself in my mind. It was a picture of a hospital room, with machines beeping away, tubes dripping with mysterious liquids, the hiss of the respirator repeating its message of the finite amount of time I would remain among the living, and the nurses doing their best to adopt a passable look of sympathy just before they checked their watches with the hope of finding it closer to the end of their shifts.

No, thank you very much.

These little ping-pong matches that went on inside my head had me vacillating every now and again, pondering the wisdom of the turn I'd taken at the fork in the road. But when I managed to wrestle the fear to the ground and regain control of my emotions, a kind of peace would spill over me that warmed me to the apex of my soul.

My approach was the right one. Of this, I was sure. And no matter the result, I was going to race ahead with the same wild abandon as the guy who grew up licking his chops at the sight of menacing, 9-foot waves precluding a Gulf storm on a windy Florida day. That guy would never have run for the safety of nearby shelter. He would have grabbed his surfboard and headed for the most intimidating wave he could find.

And even if his heart was beating faster than the pistons in an engine pushed all the way to the peg, *that* guy would be at peace.

Popeye

Rock Forest, Quebec, is just under two hours by car from Montreal, and it was a place I had to go, because a man lived there that might be able to help me. My endless research had told me so.

The man's name was Gaston Naessens, and his study of molecular-level bloodstream particles had led him to the discovery of one particular, very small constituent he had dubbed the "somatid."

Somatids, Naessens argued, were responsible for normalizing key biological functions.[30] His "Somatidian Orthobiology" was a new scientific discipline that he created, and he argued that it revealed a clear "Somatidian Cycle" that was useful for comparing somatid growth and activity between bloodstreams of healthy and diseased patients.[31] These comparisons were meaningful, he said, in part because it had allowed him to formulate a product that would help to balance immune system response against germs, viruses, and cancer.[32]

His compound 714X, which was made up of ammonium chloride, nitrate, sodium chloride, ethanol, and water[33], was designed to work by promoting immune system effectiveness against abnormal cell growth. It did this, he suggested, by making nitrogen available to neutralize cancerous cells through decreasing the thickness of the body's lymph fluid.[34]

All of this sounded a bit too complex for me to digest without gathering more information, and this is why I felt obliged to make the trek northward and visit with Mr. Naessens in person. Of course, I

---

[30] http://www.cerbe.com/index2.html
[31] http://www.cerbe.com/index2.html

[32] http://alternativecancer.us/714x.htm
[33] http://alternativecancer.us/714x.htm
[34] http://alternativecancer.us/714x.htm

was still operating under some rather unfortunate time constraints, so I didn't have luxury of putting off the trip for a few months until the snow stopped falling in Canada.

Quebec, here I come, middle of winter or not.

Picking up my rental car at the airport, chains on the tires and all, I made the drive to Rock Forest right through the teeth of a wicked snowstorm and met Gaston at his home.

Our personal interaction was somewhat limited, however. Gaston's English was bad and my French was worse, so we both relied on his son to do the translating for us. Still, I could tell that Gaston had real empathy for me and seemed genuinely interested in helping me seek a recovery. He was also very humble, not all consumed with the "God Complex" that some with abilities like his might allow themselves to fall into.

With the extra time the back-and-forth discussion took, I wound up spending most of the day there, grateful to the both of them for being so professional (and so patient) as I hammered away with a thousand questions. By the time I ran out of things to ask about, I had my instructions and enough 714X (supplied for a discount at Gaston's insistence) to get me started on the program, and I braved the weather once more for the drive back to the airport in Montreal. One restless night in a nearby hotel later, I flew back to Florida and settled in to start this new course of drug treatment.

For 21 consecutive days, I self-administered the 714X via injection. The stuff is made from things most people are apt to have in small concentrations within their bodies at any given interval, so side effects didn't really seem to be a problem for me. Leastwise, there weren't any *negative* side effects.

One by-product of taking 714X, however, was the fact that my speed and agility became greatly magnified. That is *not* what the product is designed to do; I was taking it to improve my immune system, and I firmly believe that it helped me to do exactly that. But nevertheless, 714X did indeed give me a surprising ease of movement I had never experienced in my lifetime before.

When I dispensed a regular dose (never any more than 0.5cc) just before a Kung Fu training session, I would proceed to amaze my classmates, and myself, with the swift velocity of my kicks and punches. The increase in my agility was astonishing, and although the superior military-types in the class were sometimes nearly half again my size, they all came to fear the speed I could use to whale away on them when we sparred.

Popeye, eat your heart out!

The scrappy old Sailor Man and cartoon superhero I used to watch on television at 6 years old was exactly what came to my mind. The bad guy was Bluto and Popeye would eat his spinach, get real strong real fast, and save the day by beating up the bigger, badder Bluto. In my mind, I was Popeye and 714X was my spinach.

Marco Safacu, our Master, would line up the beefcakes for me one at a time during our four-hour, Saturday sparring sessions. Inexorably, I would wear one of the guys out and Marco would make me go at another, then another, and another. Finally, he would throw me up against "Big Carl" for my last fight of the day. My nimble moves and rapid strikes would land often enough to keep Carl reeling, but whenever he scored a kick on my smaller body I wound up literally flying through the air. In addition to his brawn and his raw size, Big Carl was in the Special Forces, so he had additional expertise that gave him another advantage over me. Still, in this training arena with pads and gloves, I was about as good a match as any of us could give to Carl. And despite his success at kindly kicking my ass for me every Saturday, surprisingly we became very good friends, even though he was not the type to associate with anyone.

The rest of Saturday, by then, would be left for the trappings of the television in my apartment, as a very tired but very satisfied Johnny Delirious rested his bones upon his very tired, but very satisfying couch.

Bluto

Even if I was Popeye the Sailor Man and 714X was my spinach, Bluto was still very much alive, and no matter how hard I tried to send him sulking away after a another well-timed punch, he kept coming back for more. Just like in the cartoon.

Bluto, for me, was the virus called hepatitis C, and he was still doing his level best to destroy my liver. This really didn't seem right; I had worked hard, *really* hard to get my strength back and to use that strength to fight back with all that I could muster.

So far, though, it hadn't been enough.

Feeling confident after the latest flight of 714X injections, Kung Fu training, Zapper treatments and still maintaining an alcohol-free, nutrient-rich natural diet, I decided to take stock of how my liver was responding to all of this. I went for a blood test and the results were, well, disappointing at best. My body was simply not responding quickly enough to the course of treatment I had chosen. Yes, my liver enzyme levels had gone down *some*, but they were still too high, and they were certainly still consistent with the very things my doctors and everybody else were warning me about.

Score another one for 'ol Bluto, I guess.

It would be easy to become despondent at this point, but somehow I managed to check that emotion at the door and take out a little withdraw against all the recent strength I had deposited. Come what may, I decided that Popeye's spinach was going to have to help restore the muscle between his ears along with the ones in his arms. Popeye, I reasoned, was going to have to stay brave if he wanted to stay alive.

Rescuing myself from another episode of nearly giving up the ship entirely, I set the blood test results aside and made another promise to myself that I would respond by pushing harder for the natural cure I was seeking. I resolved that I'd play Popeye for as long as I could, resisting the urge to give up, and take my spinach and do my exercise and maybe even step up my efforts to find new therapies. That was good, that sort of thinking, and it left me with just one small problem.

    The clock was still ticking.

Fanatic

It was time to get serious now, because there simply wasn't enough time for anything else.

A $250 blood test had revealed that my "viral load" was over 5 million, which is not exactly good. Anything over 800,000 International Units per milliliter of blood is considered "high."[35] So now, there was concrete evidence that the hepatitis C was actively reproducing and infecting more and more cells in my body.[36]

Like I said, time for Delirious to get serious.

With this latest news, my appetite for finding new therapies was becoming as ferocious as my disease's attempts to take me out. Capitalizing on the benefits of being a student at Western Florida University, I put my efforts into overdrive and found myself getting kicked out of the campus library past closing time on more than one occasion.

The internet, too, had become a useful tool for searching out information quickly. But it was the era of Netscape and AOL, and much of the search engine work I did was of course limited by the amount of legacy information that was still finding its way onto the Web. In any case, I did so much reading that sometimes the paragraphs merged together into such a haze that I couldn't see the pages anymore, much less the words themselves.

All of this obsessive research uncovered a few things I was inclined to chase down, but every now and again I'd find something that caused the fog to clear away and grab my attention in full. One such discovery came in the form of several articles that focused on the benefits of oxygen therapies.

---

[35] http://www.hcvadvocate.org/hepatitis/factsheets_pdf/VIRALLOAD.pdf
[36] http://www.hcvadvocate.org/hepatitis/factsheets_pdf/VIRALLOAD.pdf

The studies I ran across suggested that viruses and bacteria cannot survive very long without a host to shield them from open air, and in particular, the hepatitis C virus could subsist for no more than four days when exposed to oxygen. With that in mind, I began to focus on therapies that were designed to maximize oxygen in the tissues of the body.

Enter the phenomenon of hyperbaric oxygen treatment.

The protocol for this treatment involves placing the patient into a hermetically sealed chamber, where he is exposed to 100% pure oxygen under increased atmospheric pressure.[37] By using pure oxygen under pressure instead of regular air (the air we breathe contains only about 21% oxygen)[38] the body's ability to repair itself can theoretically be given a significant boost.[39]

Hyperbaric oxygen treatment had been around for a long time, with some evidence suggesting it dated as far back as the 15th century.[40] The therapy was developed in modern times by the US military, and has been implemented most famously as the method by which deep-sea divers are treated for the "bends."[41] The "bends" are caused by decompression as a result of surfacing too rapidly as a diver ascends from deep waters.

With hyperbaric oxygen therapy, the bloodstream is infused with pure oxygen in a "hyper" magnified way; some studies suggest that the concentrations can increase by as much as 2,000%.[42] With this kind of intensity, and particularly when applied under increased pressure, the oxygen can reach bone and other tissue much more readily, which can lead to accelerated healing of a wide variety of afflictions.[43]

After reading as much as I could gather about this promising treatment, I found out that one of the premier places to get it was right there in my home state of Florida. It was called the Ocean Hyperbaric Oxygen Center, and it was founded by Dr. Richard Neubauer.

Next stop; Fort Lauderdale.

---

[37] http://www.oceanhbo.com/client/ohc/what.htm
[38] http://encarta.msn.com/encyclopedia_1741500785/air.html
[39] http://www.oceanhbo.com/client/ohc/what.htm
[40] http://inventors.about.com/library/inventors/blhyperbaric.htm
[41] http://inventors.about.com/library/inventors/blhyperbaric.htm
[42] http://www.oceanhbo.com/client/ohc/what.htm
[43] http://www.oceanhbo.com/client/ohc/what.htm

Over the next four weeks, I devoted myself to intensive hyperbaric oxygen therapy at Dr. Neubauer's clinic. By now, school was out for the summer so I could focus on putting what I had learned back in Pensacola to good use there in Fort Lauderdale. After reviewing my case, Dr. Neubauer scheduled 120 minute treatments that would take place six out of seven mornings for those four weeks. It was to be something of a crash course, rivaling anything the university could throw at me in my studies back home.

--

Another blood test revealed that the hyperbaric Oxygen treatments had improved my liver enzyme levels incrementally, but still not enough. The levels were still high.

It seemed like I was doing better, though. I mean, I certainly *felt* better, but my body was not recovering fast enough. Still, I was dogged in my determination to eradicate this virus, and I was going to make it happen, somehow, without the use of drug cocktails. I wanted to do it by continuing to strengthen my body, such that my immune response would take over and do the dirty work for me.

When I returned to Pensacola from Fort Lauderdale, I picked up where I left off in my research, desperately fanatic about finding more and more therapeutic ways to kick hepatitis out of my life for good. I worked voraciously on all the programs I had started, continuing with the Zapper, the 714X, the Kung Fu, and the healthy eating. All of this was giving me plenty of energy to carry out my research and my regiments, and if nothing else, the *Mello Yellow* had subsided to the point where my jaundice was not so obvious.

All of this had made me skinny, too. But that was small consolation, because by now I had to hope that dropping a few pounds was good for something more than a comfortable fit inside a rectangular, pine box.

The Rule

Quickly, now! What's the rule? It's simple, really. OK, I'll give you a hint:

*The Rule is, Never Do Anything
That Might Be Harmful to Your Body*

Up to now, with time fading away faster than a fat kid eating his second piece of cake, I had been a good boy and avoided any therapy or treatment that could be potentially harmful to the body. Since embarking upon my agenda for a natural cure, I had not yet broken the rule. And I didn't intend to do so going forward, either.

Hyperbaric oxygen was a therapy that seemed to have helped, but it could not be continued for more than 3 or 4 weeks at a time. It was a good, solid notch on the barrel of my healing gun, but I needed more.

Naturopathy seemed like a "natural" next step, so I began my study of it and looked hard at anything designed to fortify my body and exaggerate my immune response. And since I was satisfied with the experience at Dr. Neubauer's clinic, I started looking for other kinds of medical firms or hospitals that might be able to help.

I hated to admit it, but Johnny Delirious *needed* help.

Gerson Clinic

Safe and natural, that's what the Gerson Institute calls its program of organic nutrition and detoxification. When I read that, I thought, "OK, that doesn't sound like it breaks any rules."

Max Gerson developed his course of therapy way back in the 1920's. In simple terms, the regimen is designed to stimulate the body's natural ability to heal itself. It does this by working to reverse the years of exposure all of us have to toxins that we eat, drink, and breathe in our everyday lives.[44]

By executing the Gerson therapy, patients hope to capitalize on its comprehensive methods for magnifying the body's own capacity for repairing itself. The program is touted by supporters as an excellent alternative treatment for cancer and other progressive diseases. And although I didn't have cancer, the literature about Gerson especially caught my eye when I saw that their detoxification process is intended to purge the liver of toxins that have been collected over the course of a person's life.

Organic nutrition. Detoxification. Nutrient mega-dosing.
Purged liver.
Where do I sign up?

Back in Mexico, it turns out. The Gerson Institute itself is headquartered in San Diego, and the treatment center closest to the Institute just happened to be located in a small town 10 miles south of Tijuana. It's called *Playa Rosarito*.

Feeling genuinely excited about the prospects for this cleansing therapy, I called the Institute for more information, peppering the poor girl on the other end of the line with my usual ten thousand questions. The more she said, the more I liked what I heard, and by the time we

---

[44] http://www.gerson.org/g_therapy/default.asp

were finished talking I knew I wanted to be a patient at Gerson. She seemed happy to have me and eager to get me signed on, right up until she asked me who my partner for the in-patient therapy would be.

"I'll be attending by myself," I said. To which she replied that the treatments at Gerson were quite rigorous and having a partner (wife, relative, friend, etc) was a prerequisite to joining up. Not one to give up easily, I pestered the gal for a few minutes more, but she was unflappable and insistent that there were no exceptions to this rule.

This little development was a bit of a problem for me, to say the least. My family had all but disowned me, and I was sure they would view another trip to Mexico for this treatment as further evidence that I was certifiably nuts.

Delirious, if you will.

But I was convinced that the Gerson Institute was the right move, so I wouldn't let up over the next few days. I called the Institute over and over again, making a fine pest of myself until someone finally suggested I talk to Charlotte Gerson. Charlotte is the daughter of Max Gerson, who had invented the therapy back in the 1920's.

Charlotte founded the Gerson Institute in 1977, and she was still running the business now. When we talked on the phone, she was at first insistent that I find a partner to help me through the therapy. It was quite rigorous, she said, and there had not been many patients at Gerson who endured the treatment alone.

Refusing to let it go, I pushed harder and harder with Charlotte, telling her my story and painting a picture of myself that let her see the hard core guy I had become. After a few more direct questions and a lot more coaxing on my part, she finally relented and agreed to a departure from the Institute's policy.

It took some doing, but I was in.

--

San Diego was the point of departure for the Gerson Clinic I would be attending in Mexico. The Institute had a van ready to take me south of the border, and as I climbed aboard I felt apprehensive for the first time since I made the decision to sign up. That's probably because the Clinic in Mexico required cash up front. Which meant that I was about to cross the tense border with its watchful Customs &

Immigration personnel while carrying wads of $100 bills stuffed into my pockets.

Getting arrested on suspicion of being a drug dealer was definitely *not* in the Gerson brochure.

I got through the stress by thinking about God and my gratitude for being alive. I thought about how lucky I was to have this chance to go to this clinic that might help to save my life. I allowed myself a moment of satisfaction at having prevailed in the negotiating battle that would make me one of the few Gerson patients to attend without a partner. And I allowed myself an early taste of Mexican culture as I remembered the sublime sounds of Herb Alpert and the Tijuana Brass and their hit, *The Lonely Bull.*

For a moment, all my fears went away as I played that song in my head. With Herb's trumpet blasting away, I started dreaming about enchiladas, tacos, rice and beans, just like I used to enjoy during my time at the *other* Institute I attended in Mexico, under so much better circumstances than these. But the thoughts of those good times went away soon enough when I remembered that I was sick with hepatitis C, and I would no doubt be on a diet that didn't include the savory flavors of the local cuisine.

Back to reality, Johnny, there would be no thrills. There would only be hope.

--

Perhaps it's serendipity that I always seem to land on a beach.

Playa Rosarito, home to one of the best Gerson Clinics on the planet, is also home to a beautiful beach. The setting made the clinic feel like just about anything but a hospital; it was a wonderful place and patients are made to feel at home from the moment they arrive. And even though most of the Gerson patients are there for cancer treatment, even us occasional "other" disease sufferers feel welcome, too.

The clinic had a full compliment of doctors, nurses and staff, as well as teachers that educated attendees about the how's and the why's of the various treatment regimes.

There were 13 glasses of fresh fruit and vegetable juices every day. Each meal was completely organic, a perfect match for my own dining routines of late. There were more private therapies, too; high colonic coffee enemas were delivered regularly, all part of the detoxification process. Organic juices and meals were consumed in community fashion in the clinic's common dining area.

The enemas, not so much, they were in our rooms.

All of the therapy was quite demanding, which is why the Institute insists on patients having a partner to help them through it. But I figured that if I could survive Kung Fu sparring matches against Big Carl, surely I could survive the Gerson treatments. In my imagination, I was Grasshopper again, bravely lifting the scalding bronze caldron and feeling the dragons being permanently burned into the flesh of my arms.

And if I could survive all of that, then maybe I could survive hepatitis C, too.

--

We were a group of just under a dozen patients from the UK, Australia, Canada, California and Texas. I was the only one from Florida, and I was the only one without a spouse or a friend to help.

Over the four-week course of treatment, we all got to know each other well and we shared our stories freely; that in and of itself was therapy, for sure. It was also therapeutic to have the opportunity to be in such good company; my room was right next door to Roxie Roker, who played Helen Willis in the hit TV sitcom *The Jeffersons*.

Roxie was also cousin to Al Roker, the famous TV weatherman, and she was Lenny Kravitz's mother. Kravitz is a well-known rock musician and songwriter famous for hits such as *Fly Away* and *Are You Gonna Go My Way?*

Because of her own popularity and her connection with Lenny, Roxie was friends with many famous people that came to the clinic to wish her their best. Lenny himself showed up every weekend, and I got to know him pretty well as a result. I told him that he had the longest dreadlocks I'd ever seen.

Roxie was not the only "good company" that Gerson could boast about. Dr. Albert Schweitzer, for example, is quoted directly on the Institute's website[45] as follows:

---

[45] http://www.gerson.org/g_therapy/default.asp

*"I see in Dr. Gerson one
if the most eminent geniuses
in the history of medicine."*

Schweitzer was a Gerson patient at one time, and in case you've forgotten, he received the Nobel Peace Prize in 1952 for his *Reverence for Life* philosophical work.[46]

Nice to have such a famous man within the medical community actually *endorse* one treatment I was engaging.

--

Since I was not a cancer patient, my doctor allowed me the high pleasure of an occasional foray off site for a swim at the beach. Her name was Dr. Melendez, and she also allowed me to hit the local gym for a good, hard workout.

As I moved through the therapy with the same focused determination as everything else I'd tried so far, the Gerson treatment worked its wonders and I felt vibrantly alive and thoroughly cleansed all the way through to my very bones. The Mexican staff on duty performed above and beyond any hospital standard, and their processes and care to make everything right was exceptional.

Near the end of the treatment, Dr. Melendez was satisfied that I had benefited from the Gerson Therapy as much as anyone could and she allowed me a few meals at the local market to go along with my other off-site activities.

Thanks to Dr. Melendez, I got a taste of those enchiladas, rice and beans after all.

---

[46] http://en.wikipedia.org/wiki/Albert_Schweitzer

Depression

All right, so maybe I was experiencing the five stages of grief in a little different order than most.

So what?

It was my life, and I could choose to deal with my situation on my own terms, couldn't I?

Denial and acceptance of the consequences of my disease had already come and gone. Denial had passed pretty much according to Hoyle, but clearly acceptance was supposed to come much later than it had for me. Of course, the definition of just what exactly constitutes "acceptance" might differ from one person to the next.

In my case, "acceptance" just meant that I was pretty sure the doctors were right about the seriousness of my condition. I could accept the fact that my disease could very well kill me; I just wasn't ready to accept the speed with which it might do so if I followed my doctors' recommendations.

Presently, however, acceptance, anger and denial were all long gone from my mind. Now I was thinking about how my liver enzyme levels were not improving, even after the Gerson treatment. I mean, come on! My colon was squeaky clean now, I was juiced up on mega doses of high-vitamin content nutrients, I had saturated my flesh and bones with pure oxygen, and I was in the best physical condition of my lifetime. So why were my enzyme levels not improving?

It was downright depressing.

All of this natural and alternative treatment had failed to get things under complete control, and so I was depressed. Not to the point of succumbing to the "deer in the headlights" syndrome, but I was just so hopeful that after the Gerson boot camp was finished, I would see some level of progress regarding key liver functions (AGOT, SGPT), on the blood profile reports.

Maybe because I expected too much too soon, I missed the message of hope that was hidden in my latest enzyme level results. They may not have been going *down,* but they weren't going *up,* either.

Rife

Home from the Gerson Clinic in Mexico for the rest of the summer, I came back to headlines that told of another baseball strike, another Woodstock, and another round of wildfires out west, which killed 14 firefighters this time around. Most of the tidings in the newspaper were just as discouraging as the ones about my latest liver enzyme test results.

Back to the drawing board I went, with just as much energy as before, albeit with a little bit less conviction. There was depression in the wake of these liver enzyme evaluations, and there was desperation as well. With nowhere else to go, I arranged my mind into punt formation, ready to kick the ball down the field of gritty and determined research once again.

Organizing the notebooks and outlines from my earlier work, I poured through it all once more, following up here and there whenever I ran across something that got my attention. After a few hours of exhaustive reading, some notes I had made about the Rife Microscope wound up centered in my crosshairs.

Royal Raymond Rife was probably most famous for the development of an optical microscope that he claimed could observe viruses and bacteria without killing them, as was the case with the electron microscope.[47] By allowing unfettered viewing of live viruses, meaningful observations about the activity, life span, ability to reproduce, and overall strength of them could be made. The next logical conclusion is that the medical community might learn how to defeat such viruses and bacteria if it could examine them while they were still alive.

---

[47] http://www.xenophilia.com/zb0012a.htm

Rife made some conclusions of his own after using his Universal Microscope to evaluate viruses. He suggested that the microscope had revealed patterns of light unique to each type of virus, and that after experimenting with frequency oscillation directed at the virus, he could kill the organism without effecting healthy tissues in the host.[48]

In Rife's opinion, one particular virus that he studied was definitively a carcinogen. Calling this virus "Cryptocides Primordiales" (primordial hidden killer)[49], Rife proceeded to run some experiments where he injected the CP virus into 400 laboratory test animals, resulting in the creation of tumors in every one of them.[50] Then he used his frequency oscillation device on each of the test animals, and according to the story, all 400 of the tumors disappeared from the host animals.[51] Later, in a research project sponsored by the University of Southern California involving humans, Rife's treatment was purported to have led to the full recovery of an unknown number of terminal cancer patients after 130 days.[52]

There has been a lot of editorial writing and plenty of controversy surrounding Rife's claims. Many people believe that Rife was a victim of *The Establishment,* medical-community style, in much the same way as groundbreakers such as Louis Pasteur, whose ideas were ridiculed before they were accepted.

Perhaps Jonathan Swift said it best:

> "When a true genius appears in this world, you may know him by this sign: that the dunces are all in confederacy against him."

My notes regarding Rife's Universal Microscope triggered in my mind the memory of a book about Rife's work called *The Cancer Cure That Worked.* I had come across it in Dallas when I was packing up Davenport Labs for liquidation. Locating the book in one of the boxes I had brought back from Texas, I paged through it and learned

---

[48] http://www.mnwelldir.org/docs/cancer1/rife.htm
[49] http://www.mnwelldir.org/docs/cancer1/rife.htm
[50] http://www.mnwelldir.org/docs/cancer1/rife.htm
[51] http://www.mnwelldir.org/docs/cancer1/rife.htm
[52] http://www.mnwelldir.org/docs/cancer1/rife.htm

that Rife's Frequency Oscillator technology might still be commercially available.

Once again, I spent hours in front of the computer screen researching Rife's work, looking for anything I could find about his cancer treatment protocol. It turned out that there were indeed several companies selling an equivalent to Rife's treatment machine, so I picked the one that looked the most reputable and bought one. It set me back over $2,600, money I didn't have, really. But at this point, I reasoned that I wasn't just buying a machine. I was making an investment in hope.

--

Waiting for the Rife machine to be delivered would put me on pins and needles for a few days, so I concentrated furiously on using the time for more research. I continued the treatments I'd already started, including the 714X, the organic foods and juices, and of course, the Zapper.

Firing up Dr. Hulda Clark's Zapper one morning got me to thinking about some additional therapies she advocated. Returning to her website, I read about her liver and kidney cleanses, which she recommended in addition to the parasite eradication that her Zapper technology promised.

Clark cautioned visitors to her site about the proper order of these treatments, suggesting that the organ cleanses be done only after the parasite treatment. Then, for best results, she indicated that the kidney cleanse should also come before the liver flush, so that the urinary tract and bladder can handle removal of residual substances absorbed from the intestines as liver bile is pushed out.[53] Well, I was thinking that I was in good shape regarding parasites since I had been using the Zapper, but I wasn't interested in wasting time by going in order with the kidneys first and liver second. I wanted it all, and I wanted it now. So Popeye, a.k.a. Johnny Delirious, would move forward with all convenient speed and do both cleanses all at once.

--

---

[53] http://www.drclark.ch/en/cleanses_clean-ups/liver_cleanses.php

Dr. Clark's kidney cleanse calls for a comprehensive herbal mix that includes everything from Ginger, Hydrangea and Gravel root to Bearberry and Goldenrod.[54] The herb mixtures are made into teas that are consumed daily over a three week period, another reason I was going to do the kidney cleanse at the same time as the liver cleanse.

To a man without much time, three weeks is a big hunk of whatever he might have left.

For the liver, there would be Epsom salt solution, olive oil, grapefruit juice, and black walnut tincture.[55] All of this is accompanied with ornithine, an amino acid that is part of the "urea cycle," which is responsible for disposing of surplus nitrogen in the body.[56] The idea behind this liver cleanse is to rid the body of gallstones that block the body's ability to digest as effectively as it can. This, argues Dr. Clark, is the central basis of a person's overall heath and wellness.[57]

--

Midway through the one-two punch of these organ cleanses, my Rife machine arrived. Now I felt I had perhaps the most comprehensive line-up of curative weapons in my arsenal that I could possibly find:

- The 714X was still working to prevent blockage in my lymphatic fluid.
- My colon was in great shape from the detox of the coffee enemas.
- My nutrition was world class with all of the organic fruit and vegetable juices.
- The Zapper was still working on parasites.
- Garden of Life's *Primal Defense* probiotic supplement was working to fortify my natural intestinal microbiota.
- I was still training in Kung Fu and more recently had expanded into running.

---

[54] http://www.drclark.ch/cn/cleanses_clean-ups/kidney_cleanses.php
[55] http://www.drclark.ch/en/cleanses_clean-ups/liver_cleanses.php
[56] http://en.wikipedia.org/wiki/Ornithine
[57] http://www.drclark.ch/en/cleanses_clean-ups/liver_cleanses.php

In addition to all of this, I began the Rife treatment procedure as soon as I could get the machine out of the box. Bombarding my liver with oscillating frequency as directed by the Rife research, I was hoping that between the cleanses and this latest treatment, I would finally purge my liver of more than just impurities. The hepatitis C itself was my target, and I was going to shoot at it until I killed it or killed myself.

Hopefully, my aim would be true.

Anticipation

What with all of the strict dieting, exercise, detoxification, oxygenation, supplemental and electronic therapies I'd undertaken, I had completely exhausted myself.

I had exhausted all of my options as well; all except for one. It was the last thing left to do, and after all of my hard work I felt it was time.

It was time for another viral load test.

The last one, you'll recall, came back with less than stellar results. The viral load at the beginning of summer was over 5 million. Now that it was nearing the end of summer and I had engaged every beneficial alternative treatment I could find, I was hoping for some improvement beyond what my liver enzyme levels had shown.

I *really* needed some good news, for a change. This is what I was thinking as I sat shirtless at the end of the paper-covered examination table in a sterile room at West Florida Hospital.

Waiting for the nurse to knock on the door and come in with my test results was like waiting for an Inquisitor to heat a branding iron. I had poured every last bit of myself into trying to get well. It had been grueling, and thus far it had been without much in the way of rewards. Thinking about that, and thinking about what it was going to be like to die, I felt hot tears begin to well up and spill out.

It was OK for Grasshopper or Popeye to cry every now and again, wasn't it?

Wiping my eyes with the back of my forearm, I steeled myself for the worst and resolved that I would seek God's counsel no matter what the nurse had to say. Still, when the knock on the door finally came, it was hard to choke out the invitation for her to come in.

When she did, though, she had a smile on her face as she handed over the paper that contained the words I was here to see: *Viral Load: None Detected.*

There would be no stopping the tears now, but for once in a very long while, they were about something other than pain.

Top Gun

The words "None Detected" could just have easily applied to a report about how much healthy liver tissue Johnny Delirious had left. Having eradicated the hepatitis C virus completely, I was still saddled with the problem of rebuilding the 96% scar tissue that apparently still framed the condition of my liver.

Even Grasshopper needed more than just 4% of his liver, didn't he?

My vegetarian diet had clearly been instrumental in getting rid of the virus, but there was plainly not enough protein in that diet to help reconstruct hearty liver cells. The obvious conclusion I drew about that was to alter my eating habits slightly, and thus I began including organic meat and fresh fish from local markets in controlled amounts.

Drawing upon what I was learning in classes at Clayton College (where I was now studying Holistic Health Sciences) I looked at means to add protein and get my enzymes flowing through my blood in an optimized way. One such method involved adding to my daily spring water consumption, taking in up to a full gallon per day. The water assisted with enzyme flow through the bloodstream, a positive move for sure, but again not enough to make the kind of impact I was looking for.

The real trick at this stage was to find a way to make proteases (which are enzymes that digest protein) to act as scavengers[58] for the damaged protein cells that were now so abundant in my liver. In effect, the protease enzymes could help me by literally *eating* the scar tissue that was rendering 96% of my liver ineffective.

---

[58] http://www.enzymeessentials.com/HTML/proteases.html

Would clean water and a little bit of fish do all that for me? Unfortunately. . . not.

The last critical piece of the scar tissue puzzle was to force enzymes into all of my tissues as fast as I could make them flow. And the best way to do *that*, as far as my classes at Clayton and my research could tell me, was to maximize my cardiovascular exercise.

Run, Johnny, run!

These were the words that came to the forefront of my mind. I would have to focus my physical training on a new regimen, one that included as much running as I could possibly tolerate. And being Johnny Delirious, who so far in his life had done few things in a half-baked way, I decided that there was really only one kind of running that would be suitable for me.

Marathons.

This time, I wouldn't need to sit in front of the computer for long hours dedicated to research. Everything anyone could ever want to know about marathons could be found right here in Pensacola, where the official marathon of the US Navy was held every year. It was called the Blue Angel Marathon, and I knew the moment I decided to start running that I would enter the one coming up later in the year.

So now, it was time to hang up my Grasshopper hat and trade it in for one that looked a lot more like something a Naval officer might wear. It was time to say goodbye to Kung Fu for now. It was time to become a Top Gun in the US Navy Marathon.

--

Seventy-two miles a week was the minimum recommended dose of running that participants in the Navy Marathon needed to be sure they were ready. Running 5-6 miles here and there was a very different proposition than going for 26 miles straight, so you really have to prepare your body to be able to handle the stresses and fatigue you're asking it to endure in a marathon.

I was as determined to be ready as I had been about anything else, and I saw the marathon itself as something of a holy grail to reach for as I pursued better health through the grind of the training. So train I did, hard and fast, choosing to view the experience in much the same way as I had my fight to eliminate hepatitis C from my body.

It was to be a pull-out-all-the-stops adventure, just like the natural healing approach I'd taken to battle my disease.

--

When I wasn't running or studying, I spent my free time at Everman's Natural Foods Co-op, where I was still doing a lot of volunteering. My work there allowed me to enjoy a discount on the organic groceries that were still such a vital part of my overall program, but there were higher reasons I chose to remain so involved.

By now, many people in the area considered me a minor celebrity since they were aware of my recent triumph over hepatitis C. My studies at Clayton and completion of several Naturopathy certification programs had led to appearances on radio and TV to discuss nutrition and natural health programs. Everman's itself offered wellness seminars, and I had met a lot of locals through the Co-op who had ideas about good health that meshed well with my own.

At the urging of Co-op members who knew my story, I wound up starting a support group to share my experiences for the benefit of hepatitis sufferers. As word spread around a bit, the ranks of the group swelled to the point that some meetings had over 40 participants. There was a lot of good momentum, and the vast majority of the discussions were productive.

Inevitably, most of the group members found it more than just a little difficult to make the kinds of changes in their lives that I was advocating. While I never stood up there and recommended things like Rife machines or Zappers, I did promote the importance of an organic diet, detoxification, liver cleanses and of course, a complete departure from alcoholic beverages.

There were things about the support group that were not always rewarding, such as the severe demands upon my time, but by far the worst part of it was dealing with the spouses of loved ones who didn't make it. In my active time with the group, there were several people who just didn't want to go the extra mile to aid in their own recoveries, and so they wound up taking their obstinate attitudes right down with them to the grave.

Obstinate or not, the passing of a fellow support group member was never easy to swallow. Even harder was the uncomfortable occasion where I'd see the widow of a recent victim shopping alone in Everman's, her thoughts no doubt centering on resentment that Johnny Delirious should survive hepatitis C and their own spouse should not. Worse yet, I couldn't help thinking many of those widows knew deep down that their spouses hadn't done their best, failing their families and themselves along the way. And now, here we see Johnny Delirious, still alive and kicking and saying all of the same things their loved ones hadn't listened to when they were alive.

That's one heck of an "I told you so," if you get what I mean.

It was precisely that sort of image that I wanted to avoid, so I never pushed it with anyone in the group, and certainly never pushed it with someone whose spouse hadn't survived.

The experience of watching people die like that made me more and more focused on my own healing. I figured I'd better do my level best to practice what I was preaching, so I threw myself solidly into the wellness programs I had undertaken thus far.

With the Spring water and vegetables, I added enzymes, organic meat and running; lots and lots of running.

--

The night before the BAM, short for Blue Angels Marathon, the Navy arranged a dinner and had the participating runners as guests. The setting was the Naval Air Station Officer's Club, and there would be spaghetti and salad on the menu.

This was to be my first marathon, and like many other attendees at the dinner, I was thinking that spaghetti was the perfect recipe for stocking up on carbohydrates before the race. Intent on maximizing my intake, I went up to the serving station for another helping of pasta, and there she was.

One of the most beautiful women I had ever seen was standing near the food line, having a peek at the salad bar. She was a cross between Diana Ross at her peak in the 70's and Beverly Peele, one of the hottest supermodels of the 1990's. What she saw in me I will never know, but there she was, eyeing me up and down after she apparently got bored with gazing at the lettuce.

A full Navy Captain, beautiful in every way, and a flight surgeon in the Air Medical Corps to boot. When I caught her looking at me, I was tempted to find a microphone and break into song, belting out *"You've Lost that Loving Feeling"* just like Tom Cruise and Anthony Edwards in the movie.

Engage, Maverick! Engage!

I walked over to this khaki and service medal-adorned vision and proceeded to invite her to sit at my table. We talked for awhile and things seemed to be going along nicely, quite to the point where she indicated she wanted to meet me after the race the next day. "I'll be waiting for you at the finish line," she said.

That was just about the time another officer came sidling up to the table. This one was a man. Rather a *big* one. And he really, really wanted to know just what I thought I was doing by talking to this girl.

Like many of the officers at the club on this Friday night, he had been drinking too much and was evidently very keen on the idea of forcing me to forget Top Gun and start thinking Grasshopper all over again. My Kung Fu wasn't forgotten, but it was sure to be a bit rusty after abandoning it in favor of all the running. With that in mind, I wasn't all that jazzed up about dusting off my kick-and-punch routine just now.

Telling this fine gentleman that I had never met this girl before tonight did nothing to quell his anger. He was more interested in a fight, and he stoked things along by telling me in no uncertain terms to stay away from this girl, whether I knew her or not. He kind of took a step closer when he said that. Frankly, his breath would've smelled better if he'd just eaten the hind end out of a dead skunk.

Oh boy, here we go, Mr. Delirious. Are we up for a little bare knuckles on the eve of your first big marathon?

Here I was, minding my own business just moments ago, and now I was finding myself right in the middle of a jealousy game that I wanted no part of at all. Thankfully, just before things tilted out of control, the officer's buddies showed up to calm him down and pull him away. They all disappeared into the crowd, leaving me alone once again with the ebony beauty that had caused all this trouble in the first place.

"Trouble" is exactly what I told her she was, but she didn't care and told me she'd see me after the run tomorrow just the same. "Don't worry about him, he has to take orders from me," she said.

Unsure of how much this pretty creature had to drink herself, I wrote it all off and stole away from the officer's club, intent on getting some rest before the early start of the race in the morning.

--

Driving across the Pensacola Bridge on the way back home, I was thinking about how I'd just been mired in some soap opera drama when I noticed I needed to stop for gas.

Stepping inside to pay the cashier, I bumped into the wife of one of the hepatitis support group members. When she saw me she started to cry. Her husband had just died the day before and she really needed to talk. Right now, please, and just a little over eight hours before I had to leave the house for the marathon in the morning.

I did my best to shut down a pang of selfishness as I thought about how early I needed to get up in the morning. Running in a marathon is a major physical event for someone that is completely healthy, much less a person like me with a barely functioning liver. So for me, adequate rest on this night was not just a good idea; it was critical to avoiding potentially serious medical consequences. But of course I could not brush this poor woman off or ignore her, so I agreed to talk with her right then and there at the gas station.

She had hepatitis C as well, so in addition to the strife over losing her husband she had her own well-being to worry about. I did my best to comfort her and bring her an ounce or two of hope, and by the time we wrapped it up, it was well after midnight and I really needed to get some rest.

When the alarm woke me up in the morning, I had only clocked four hours of sleep, and now my thoughts turned to an ounce of hope for myself. Hope that I could still *finish* this race, my dreams of turning in a competitive time all but washed away with the support group lady's tears just four hours ago.

--

Nothing will get the heart of a true patriot beating faster than the sight of the Blue Angel jetfighters screaming across the horizon at several hundred miles an hour. With a low flight deck and the sound of the afterburners suspended until the jets passed, the adrenaline surge I felt at the starting line of the race was unreal.

Now the worry about so little rest was gone from my mind. As the crack of the starting pistol signaled the launch of the race, I surged ahead with the force of an F-18A Hornet. I was Maverick in Top Gun all over again, complete with the pretty officer who would be there to greet me when I blazed across the finish line in record time.

My own afterburners, however, started to flame out a little by the time I crossed the five mile marker. Lost in my thoughts about the gorgeous flight surgeon who wanted to see me later, I came back to reality quickly when I remembered the words of the male officer who'd challenged me the night before. If I ignored his warning and met with this girl anyway, it was likely that 'ol Johnny Delirious would have to face a beating from the Navy Squids who would no doubt be out to get him. That was a sobering thought, and now the whole Tom Cruise thing was starting to wear a little thin.

Five miles later, Rudolph Jun passed me by as if I were going backwards. Jun, who was from my home town of Fort Walton Beach, would go on to finish first in the race with an excellent time of two hours, twenty minutes.

Me? I was just hoping to finish at all.

At mile marker 13, only halfway through, I was thinking about the support group again, and the despondent woman who lost her husband just two days ago. Even the passing of her spouse had not been enough to get her to swear off the alcohol. How can I help them all? How can I save them from themselves, I wondered as I ran.

Five more miles, and the exhaustion was so profound that I realized I could only help myself. My ego thus far had not helped me at all. In these first 18 miles of the marathon, I had gone from winner to loser, ambitious to realist, and crusader to victim.

Crossing the 20 mile marker some time later, I simply had to blank everything out. I just pounded my feet into the pavement, enduring the slog of the last six miles in dizzy cloud that left me blind to anything but the next white line on the road.

It was excruciating.

I finished nevertheless, but I had to suffer the indignity of the good-looking Naval officer's blow-off at the end of the race. She was nowhere to be found. Maybe she got tired of waiting.

I did manage to narrowly miss an indignity of another kind. I avoided turning in my personal worst time; there was at least some small consolation in that. Still, my performance was a far cry from my previous marathon training runs, where I sometimes turned in times that were under four hours. This one, however, had covered five hours and eighteen minutes, putting me just two runners away from dead last in my age group.

Not exactly supersonic jetfighter stuff, but considering everything I'd faced over the last year, I was happy with it even so.

Liver = Life

They call it the liver because it keeps us *living*. The heart does that too, of course. That's why the first thing they check in the emergency room is always the patient's blood pressure.

From my perspective, though, maybe the heart is just a tad bit overrated. Yes, without the function of the beating heart to supply blood to all of our bodily systems, we all go straight to the fossil farm. But the without the liver, we fall asleep in the narrow bed just as fast, don't we? Look no further than the fact that the heart delivers 25% of the blood it pumps directly to the liver after every single heartbeat.[59]

The liver has literally hundreds of chemical functions and conversions it must perform every minute we breathe. That's more than any of our other organs, which may well explain why the liver is so much bigger then the rest of them.

As the body's primary "filter," the liver cleanses over a liter of blood every minute. It is also responsible for producing over a quart of digestive bile every day, as well as around 4,000 enzymes, half which the medical community has yet to fully understand.[60]

Just two of the liver's critical functions, the balancing of sugars and electrolytes on a moment to moment basis, enables our blood to carry balanced nutrition to the heart and brain. Without that process, the heart itself couldn't function properly, resurrecting the argument about which organ is more important in the first place.

The liver truly makes life possible. When it is in balance, our bodies are in balance. When it is not, we simply cannot be considered healthy.

---

[59] www.associatedcontent.com/article/213047/the_livers_importance_in_the_human.html
[60] http://anabolicminds.com/forum/exercise-science/1124-importance-your-liver.html

There is more to good health than just a healthy liver, no doubt. Psychologists make a good case that mental well being is often the difference between survival or death in patients with equivalent afflictions. A reasonable person knows that a good attitude is crucial to keeping us out of trouble both physically and mentally. Attitude, by its natural extension, adds up to conviction, principle, will power and ultimately, *life* if we apply it to doing whatever is necessary to live.

We know that the liver is indispensable in our lives. Attitude is, too. Having the right attitude about doing what is best for your liver is, in the end, one key way to avoid the end itself.

Or at least postpone it, anyway.

I only wished that more of the people in my hepatitis support group could understand that concept and *live* by it to a higher degree. I remember thinking that very thing the moment I saw the gal who had lost her husband that night before the Blue Angels Marathon.

I saw her again the night after the race, too. This time, she was drunk and belligerent; taking out the bitterness at her husband's passing on me. It was as if she blamed me for his very death, and even for her own situation, as she was sure she was going to join him very soon as a result of her own hepatitis C. Unfortunately she was probably right, because she was taking out her anger not only on me, but also on her liver through the abuse she was dealing it with her drinking.

After I broke away from her, I asked myself, *"Why are people so stubborn?"* Why couldn't they accept the fact that having a degenerative liver disease meant that you had to change your habits if you didn't want to die?

Wait just a second, though. I too had been stubborn, hadn't I? Yet my stubbornness had led, in an odd way, to me being alive and very healthy. The stubbornness of others had led to poor health and now some of them were very much dead.

Dead or alive, those of us in that support group were all deviants from the recognized mainstream. We all had a non-mainstream disease. But those in the group that remained "mainstream" through their conventional lifestyle choices watched those choices lead to a shorter life's journey. My holistic health choices were leading to a longer journey, such that I was running in marathons and indeed, having the strength for just about any kind of race that life could throw my way.

Yes, we were all deviants, I suppose. But maybe we should allow for the idea that there are negative deviants and positive deviants. Surely in the case of Johnny Delirious, by deviating from conventional thinking in order to survive, he had become a *Positive Deviant* in his own right.

Riders on the Storm

It was sad. Too many of the people I was working with in the support group would come to our meetings one week, only to see them gone forever in the next. For most of these people, the reports from the doctors told them they would die, and not only did they *believe* it, in some cases it seemed like they'd actually given their consent. Accordingly, many in the group were really just there for their own version of the proverbial Hail Mary. They had long ago surrendered to the idea that they were dying and the support group was nothing more than a last resort. In short, they were waiting it out, much like a huddle of shivering refugees sitting in the corner of a hurricane shelter. They weren't doing anything but waiting, and hoping that the foreboding rain would simply pass.

They were riders on the storm, and all of them were different. Hepatitis, you see, is an equal opportunity employer. We had more than 300 support group members over the time that I was involved, and they came from all walks of life. And for these riders on the storm, there would be no reprieve; almost all of them were swept away with the fury of the winds that this cruel disease could unleash.

But in our group, there were a select few that had made the choice to step away from the sanctuary of shelter and venture out toward a more proactive path. One was a Vietnam Vet who had become a mailman upon his return from the war. Another was a flight attendant who worked for Delta Airlines. There was a billionaire's wife who drove a brand new Bentley, a fearless fisherman, a natural bodybuilder, and a practicing registered nurse. There was even a doctor, who with the RN wanted to remain anonymous for fear that their acceptance of my ideas would bring scorn from their colleagues in medicine.

There were eight of them in total. The G-8, I called them. Besides me, they were the only ones who persevered and got free from the grip of the virus. They, like me, had simply reasoned that in order to get well, a decision to do so had to be made.

After a time, I made another kind of decision, this one a lot harder than the ones about my choices for treatment. I decided to break away from the group, realizing that I couldn't help everybody. Check that; I really couldn't help *anybody* that didn't first want to help themselves. I had never pushed my ideas upon anyone, I had never charged a penny for the information I shared, and I never meant to play doctor. I merely told my story, and hoped that it might help at least a few people win the race against hepatitis C.

Johnny Delirious already had. For me, the hepatitis marathon was over.

Walk The Line

"Fourteen years."

Few words I had ever spoken were delivered more proudly than these two simple ones. Understandable, since I was still here to say them.

He was only trying to ask an uncomplicated question, one that I was admittedly more than just a little eager to answer. But he asked, and I answered. I was going to be one of the lucky ones, thank you very much.

It had been *fourteen years* since the Director of Gastroenterology at University Medical in Jackson, MS had told me I'd be dead in eight months. Yep, dead in less than a year if I didn't accept her advice and get myself signed on to the liver transplant waiting list. Yet here I was, still alive in 2006, where a different doctor in Fort Lauderdale was asking me about my health history in preparation for an exam.

The doctor in question was originally from Bolivia, and he was a liver specialist with expertise in cirrhosis. He was performing a standard evaluation recognized in medicine as the "does the liver quiver?" test, which is designed to give a reliable estimate of how much of the liver was healthy, and how much of it was scar tissue. It is non-invasive (not like a biopsy would be) but when administered by a trained technician, it still serves as a dependable method for assessing the state of a person's liver.

After reviewing the reports and the blood test results from my past, the doctor could not believe the comparison between what they were in 1992 and what they were now. Here in 2006, there was no evidence at all of antibodies to hepatitis C in my blood. Put another way, any doctor looking at that report would have no idea that I'd ever had hepatitis in my entire lifetime, much less come to the conclusion that I had it now.

Incredulous at the story those reports were telling him, the Doc proceeded with the physical exam. Designed to determine the level of scar tissue proliferation, the "does the liver quiver?" exam is sometimes referred to as the "thump" test. The patient is directed to lie on his back, while the doctor presses on the body with one hand in the areas nearby the liver. With the other hand, a swift jab is delivered just above the liver, and the amount of "wiggle" that is felt in the body is an indication of the liver's healthiness. In the case of a patient with significant scar tissue, there will be very little wiggle. For a patient with a healthy liver, the doctor will detect a greater amount of "liver quiver."

Well, my liver was quivering all right. The doctor couldn't believe it, so he must have made me flip between lying on my back and lying on my stomach at least a dozen times. He thumped my liver again and again, and with each successive thrust it told him it was quite jiggly and happily alive. His reaction was very satisfying; he had a look on his face that probably would've matched the one Christopher Columbus wore when he finally reached land.

This was a highly welcome difference from the thump tests I'd experienced back in 1992. Several different doctors had performed the exam on me in the days before my diagnosis, and when the last one took her shot at my stiffened liver, she said "I don't feel anything either. Do a biopsy."

No need for any biopsies now. This doctor said as much, proclaiming that I had the liver of a man in his twenties. Not bad for crusty old guy of 53, if I do say so myself.

As I write these words right now, my fingers fly across the keys of my laptop like I'm moving in another dimension. Ever since I started the liver cleanses that washed away my gallstones, there have been many days where I felt like I was sprinting through air and everyone else was moving in slow motion, bogged down in thick molasses. On the occasions where my peers were keeping up, it seemed they needed the erratic high that only mega-doses of caffeine could give them.

Jumping beans, that's what they were. They made unsustainable, fast movements in tiny circles that kept getting smaller and smaller, doing little in the way of meaningful work and ultimately spewing a bunch of hot air. The whole concept kind of reminds me of *The Wild, Wild West,* one of my favorite shows growing up.

In one particular episode, James West had to battle a criminal mastermind by the name of Doctor Lovelace. With the help of a special formula, Lovelace could move so fast that he'd be invisible to the naked eye, allowing him to rob banks and create all manner of havoc against the show's hero. The key ingredient to the formula was diamonds, so the cycle of Lovelace drinking the potion and using the resulting fast-forward mode to steal more diamonds was self-perpetuating.

While I had never stolen diamonds or anything else, as a matter of fact it sometimes felt as if I was just as quick as Dr. Lovelace. That kind of speed can make a man impatient, so I've had to keep myself in check many times when dealing with people who seemed like they were stuck in the mud. Everyone just seems to keep getting older all around me, even the ones that were born long after I was.

This point seemed to really hit home at both my 20 and 30 year reunions, where I was healthy enough to attend each of them despite being diagnosed with terminal hepatitis C. Some from my generation were not so lucky. The ups and downs of life were real; they were right in my face all the time, reminding me of just how much stranger truth is than fiction.

But fiction can help to tie the mysteries of life into neat little packages. Whether I was Grasshopper, Popeye or Top Gun, the people around me thought I was Delirious to the very end. Many times, 'ol Johnnie was the only one who thought he would make it, the rest of the people in his life dismissing him as a complete lunatic.

I guess I can accept that. And I guess that if the odds are stacked against you in such a way that all hope seems entirely lost, you have to get a little crazy if you are going to try and beat 'em. I hope the people in my life can understand *that*. Because after all is said and done, Johnny Delirious was only trying to walk the line, no matter whether he was going to do it for eight months or fourteen years or God willing, much, much longer yet.

Inside Job

Today, I run a mile and a half every other morning, and when I'm not running I'm off to Gold's Gym for a full body workout. And every evening brings a brisk, two mile walk before I settle in for the rest of the night.

The AARP sends me junk mail now, but I'll bet I'm one of the very few in that age group that isn't on a single prescription medicine. At least 90% of what I eat is cooked by me at home, and more than 90% of it is still organic.

The four times I've been back to the doctor in the last 10 years have not been very enlightening. For the bargain price of $180.00, he has told me that I am just fine and in very good health every time. As much as I like to hear that, I can think of a few things I'd rather spend the money on.

Our world today is really no different than it was for me during the years of Hepatitis High. No one likes the President. No one likes the war we're in. Our brothers, sisters, sons and daughters are being killed in a land far away from home. Jobs are hard to find, gas prices are too high, and the economy is depressed and unstable. There is still just as much political and racial turmoil today as there was in the times of my youth.

But there is one important difference from the years in my past and my time here on Earth today. Now, I refuse to get depressed about the things in the world that I cannot change. My running today is not about desperation like it was when I was fighting my disease. Today, I am not literally *running for my life,* I'm just running to keep it healthy and whole.

If all that I have been through had left me with nothing else, I would be thrilled to say that it has taught me the most important thing

I believe a person should know. It taught me that happiness and security does not come from a political climate or the whims of the hour in society. It comes from the *inside* of all of us. Happiness is a choice that *you* make, not one that everybody else makes for you.

Take it from me, Johnny Delirious; when you are healthy, you are happy. When you are truly happy, you are healthy. There is no outside influence that can give you your happiness or your health. It is really up to you, and it really is an inside job.

What's inside of me now is much simpler than what our world tries to sell us as the essential ingredients of joy. What's inside of me now is good health, God in my life, and the self-assurance that both are with me for every step that I take.

This is just a small part of Johnny's adventurous life. For more information about Johnny Delirious, his other biographies, lab tests, resume, news, etc., please go to www.johnnydelirious.com

NOTES

NOTES

NOTES

NOTES

NOTES

NOTES

NOTES

Johnathan needs a new liver

NOTES

NOTES

NOTES

NOTES

NOTES

NOTES

NOTES

NOTES

NOTES

NOTES

NOTES

(817) 287-8027 cell

Aug, Wen,
Johnathon needs his teeth done, he's deathly afair of the Dentist ~~Deptall~~ hopefully he's happy in his new house,
He's not as ~~Big~~ Big!